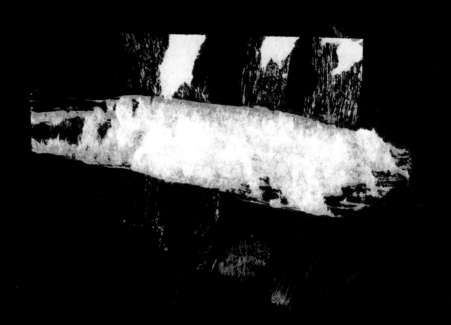

Esophagus and Stomach

Requisites in Gastroenterology
Anil K. Rustgi (ed.)

Books in the series:

Volume 1: Esophagus and Stomach, David A. Katzka, David C. Metz (eds)
Volume 2: Small and Large Intestine, Gary R. Lichtenstein, Gary D. Wu (eds)
Volume 3: Hepatobiliary Tract and Pancreas, K. Rajender Reddy,
          William B. Long (eds)
Volume 4: Endoscopy and Gastrointestinal Radiology, Gregory G. Ginsberg, Michael
          L. Kochman (eds)

Commissioning Editor: *Rolla Couchman*
Project Development Manager: *Hilary Hewitt*
Project Manager: *Alan Nicholson*
Illustration Manager: *Mick Ruddy*
Designer: *Andy Chapman*

The Requisites in

Gastroenterology

Anil K. Rustgi MD (ed.)
Chief, Division of Gastroenterology
University of Pennsylvania School of Medicine
Philadelphia, PA
USA

Volume 1: Esophagus and Stomach

Edited by
David C. Metz, MD
Professor of Medicine
Co-director, Gastroenterology Motility and
  Physiology Program
Division of Gastroenterology
University of Pennsylvania School of
Medicine
Philadelphia, PA
USA

David A. Katzka, MD
Associate Professor of Medicine
Co-director, Gastroenterology Motility and
  Physiology Program
Division of Gastroenterology
University of Pennsylvania School of
Medicine
Philadelphia, PA
USA

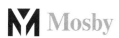 Mosby

An Imprint of Elsevier Limited
Edinburgh • London • New York • Oxford • Philadelphia • St Louis • Sydney • Toronto 2003

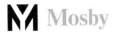 Mosby

An imprint of Elsevier Limited

© 2003, Elsevier Limited. All rights reserved.

First published 2003

ISBN 0-3230-1886-6

British Library Cataloguing in Publication Data
A catalogue record for this book is available from the British Library

Library of Congress Cataloging in Publication Data
A catalog record for this book is available from the Library of Congress

Note
Medical knowledge is constantly changing. As new information becomes available, changes in treatment, procedures, equipment and the use of drugs become necessary. The editors, contributors and the publishers have taken care to ensure that the information given in this text is accurate and up to date. However, readers are strongly advised to confirm that the information, especially with regard to drug usage, complies with the latest legislation and standards of practice.

Printed in the UK

The
Publisher's
policy is to use
**paper manufactured
from sustainable forests**

Contents

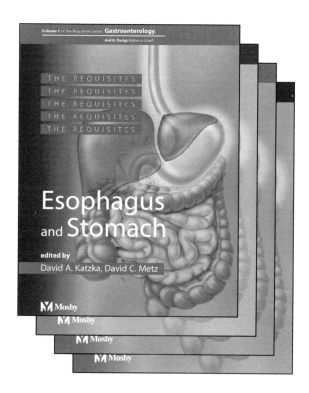
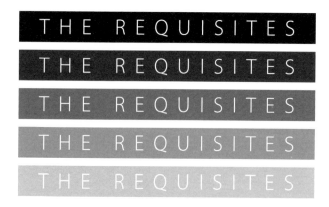

Series Foreword

This exciting and innovative *Requisites in Gastroenterology* series takes a broad-based and fundamental approach to the pathophysiology, diagnosis and management of gastrointestinal, hepatic and pancreatic diseases and disorders. The series is divided into 4 inter-related volumes, each of which in turn is edited by nationally and internationally renowned editors who are supported by excellent contributors. The contributors represent a breadth of disciplines and expertise, and are drawn from a number of different institutions and academic medical centers. At the same time, the University of Pennsylvania provides a 'home' base for the series, and indeed, its gastroenterology, surgery, radiology and pathology departments have been a foundation for clinical care, teaching and investigation for several generations.

Volume 1 deals with diseases and disorders of the esophagus and stomach, edited by Drs David Katzka and David Metz. Volume 2 covers small and large intestinal diseases and disorders, edited by Drs Gary Lichtenstein and Gary Wu. Volume 3 delineates hepatobiliary and pancreatic diseases and disorders, edited by Drs Rajender Reddy and William Long. Finally, Volume 4, edited by Drs Gregory Ginsberg and Michael Kochman, brings together the important diagnostic and therapeutic modalities of endoscopy, interventional endoscopy and radiological imaging that are of direct relevance to topics covered in Volumes 1, 2 and 3. While each volume is self-sufficient, all volumes provide the reader with a focused, cohesive and integrated view of the principles and practice of gastroenterology, hepatology and pancreatology. Each volume is well illustrated and contains tables and figures that highlight salient features of different topics. Of note, boxes are provided that encapsulate key information covered in each chapter. These collective features are meant to assist the reader. The references are pivotal ones from the literature, and are not meant to be exhaustive.

In the evolution of this series, our collective thinking was to target the audience of medical students, residents, gastrointestinal fellows, allied health professionals (nurses, nurse practitioners, physician assistants), and those physicians (gastroenterologists, hepatologists, oncologists, surgeons, pathologists, radiologists) who require overviews for certifying examinations. The series is unique in the library of books that span the discipline of gastroenterology. The reader will find the volumes 'user-friendly' and will be imparted with expert knowledge and insights, making this an engaging overview and refresher course. We hope and trust that we will succeed in this mission.

The volumes that form the kernel of this series were profoundly influenced on the one hand by students, residents and fellows, and on the other hand, by the pioneering advances of T. Grier Miller, Thomas Machella, Frank Brooks, Sidney Cohen, Richard McDermott, Peter Traber and Ed Raffensperger. It is to these past and future leaders to whom I wish to give my special gratitude.

Anil K. Rustgi, MD
Editor-in-Chief

Preface

It has been an exciting and fulfilling experience for us to work on the first volume of the *Requisites in Gastroenterology*, which deals with the esophagus and stomach. A major aim of this series is to provide algorithms and tables that allow physicians to generate useful differential diagnoses and management plans for their patients. Key references are included for readers who require more in-depth discussion on disease pathogenesis or the underlying information that was used to derive our algorithmic approach. We hope our chapters are presented in an easy-to-read manner.

The chapters in this volume are broadly arranged by organ system: the esophagus and the stomach. Gastroesophageal reflux disease (GERD) is a disease of increasing importance and significance. It is the most common reason for patients with esophageal disease to present for medical care, although it is generally an outpatient condition managed by primary care physicians. The chapter on other causes of esophagitis focuses primarily on infectious esophagitis, which is also of increasing relevance, especially in immuno-suppressed persons. An entire chapter is devoted to Barrett's Esophagus, a serious complication of GERD. Although esophageal motility disorders are relatively uncommon, we felt it necessary to include such a chapter to familiarize physicians with the approach to non-structural abnormalities of gastrointestinal function. We also felt it necessary to devote a full chapter to transfer dysphagia because these patients commonly present to gastroenterologists who must distinguish between esophageal and supra-esophageal causes for dysphagia in order to permit appro-

priate patient workup and management. We included a chapter on rings, webs, stenoses, and diverticula to cover structural abnormalities of the esophagus, which require special attention in general clinical management. The last chapter, on esophageal cancer, was another important condition which we felt deserved a dedicated chapter.

The first gastric chapter deals with *H. pylori* gastritis, the major infection of the stomach. Although *H. pylori* is a specific cause of peptic ulcer disease, there are other causes which are covered separately. Motility disorders of the stomach are discussed to highlight the difference between structural and functional foregut disease states. Nonulcer dyspepsia is also highlighted. Although the management of foreign bodies of the gastrointestinal tract almost always requires specialist consultation, there are diagnostic and management considerations that are important from a primary care perspective. The final chapter on gastric cancer, gastric lymphoma, and carcinoids of the stomach raises important epidemiologic issues. Although gastric cancer appears to be declining in frequency worldwide, it remains a major population threat; carcinoids are becoming more clinically important because of the ubiquitous use of proton pump inhibitors; and gastrointestinal lymphoma, though rare compared to other sites of primary lymphoma, is a major cause within the gastrointestinal tract.

We hope that this collection of chapters on the esophagus and stomach provide our readers with a general approach to the diagnosis and management of patients with upper gastrointestinal complaints.

This book would not have been possible without the overseeing guidance of the series editor, Dr. Anil Rustgi, whom we wish to thank. We would also like to thank the editorial staff of Elsevier as well as our chapter contributors, for whom we have great respect. Finally, we would also like to thank our respective families.

David C. Metz, MD
David A. Katzka, MD

Contributors

Faten N. Aberra MD, MSCE
Division of Gastroenterology
University of Pennsylvania School of Medicine
Philadelphia, PA
USA

Michelle Beilstein MD
Division of Gastroenterology
University of Pennsylvania School of Medicine
Philadelphia, PA
USA

Patricia Dooley CCC-SLP
Division of Audiology and Speech
Department of Otolaryngology, Head and
   Neck Surgery
University of Pennsylvania School of Medicine
Philadelphia, PA
USA

David A. Katzka MD
Associate Professor of Medicine
Co-Director, Gastroenterology Motility and
   Physiology Center
Division of Gastroenterology
University of Pennsylvania School of Medicine
Philadelphia, PA
USA

David E. Loren MD
Division of Gastroenterology
University of Pennsylvania School of Medicine
Philadelphia, PA
USA

David C. Metz MD
Professor of Medicine
Co-Director, Gastroenterology Motility and
   Physiology Center
Division of Gastroenterology
University of Pennsylvania School of Medicine
Philadelphia, PA
USA

Natasha Mirza MD, FACS
Department of Otolaryngology, Head and Neck
   Surgery
University of Pennsylvania School of Medicine
Philadelphia, PA
USA

Cesar Ruiz MA, CCC-SLP
Division of Audiology and Speech
Department of Otolaryngology, Head and Neck
   Surgery
University of Pennsylvania School of Medicine
Philadelphia, PA
USA

Janak N. Shah MD
Division of Gastroenterology
University of Pennsylvania School of
   Medicine
Philadelphia, PA
USA

Debra G. Silberg MD, PHD
Assistant Professor of Medicine
Director, Morphology Core Facility
Division of Gastroenterology
University of Pennsylvania School of
   Medicine
Philadelphia, PA
USA

John C. Sun MD
Division of Gastroenterology
University of Pennsylvania School of Medicine
Philadelphia, PA
USA

Yu-Xiao Yang MD, MSCE
Division of Gastroenterology
University of Pennsylvania School of Medicine
Philadelphia, PA
USA

Dedication

Dr Katzka dedicates this book to Margie, Emma and Will.

Dr Metz dedicates this book to Cyndie, Zoe and Tyler for enduring his frequent absences and long hours.

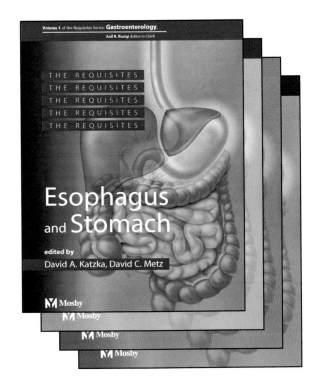
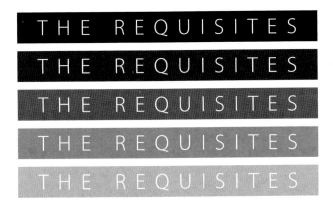

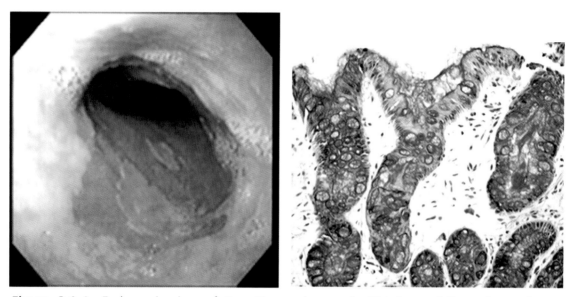

Figure 3.1 A. Endoscopic view of Barrett's esophagus. B. Histology of Barrett's esophagus, highlighting goblet cells with alcian blue staining, × 200. (see p. 41)

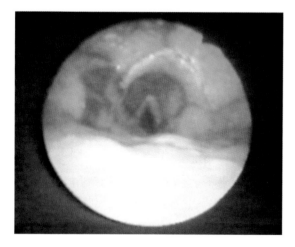

Figure 5.10 An endoscopic view as seen during the FEES procedure. Pooling is observed at the piriform sinuses. (see p. 82)

Chapter 1

Gastroesophageal Reflux Disease

David A. Katzka and David C. Metz

CHAPTER OUTLINE

Introduction

In national surveys up to 40 per cent of adults have had heartburn. It is not surprising then that proton pump inhibitors account for the most commonly prescribed medications in the world. Furthermore, authors of recent landmark articles have not only reported epidemiologically associated adenocarcinoma of the esophagus and gastroesophageal reflux but have additionally demonstrated that the incidence of esophageal adenocarcinoma is rising exponentially in this country. In fact, the incidence of adenocarcinoma of the esophagus is increasing more rapidly than any other internal malignancy. With these types of data, it is not surprising that gastroesophageal reflux disease (GERD) has received considerable attention lately both in the lay and medical press. Never before has knowledge of this disease become so imperative to the physician.

Pathophysiology

In the etiology of gastroesophageal reflux, dysfunction of the lower esophageal sphincter (LES) plays the main role. Normally, the LES acts as a barrier to the reflux of acid from the stomach into the esophagus by acting as a high-pressure zone between the lower pressures of the proximal esophagus and distal stomach, which it separates. Its pressure is strong enough to prevent higher gastric pressures, caused by activities such as straining and increasing abdominal pressure, from overcoming this barrier. On the other hand, the control of the LES must be finely tuned to allow it to relax and open for a long enough time for the passage of food with deglutition, but not so long that reflux occurs. When there is a dysfunction of either baseline tone or prolonged or frequent LES opening, the patient is then predisposed to gastroesophageal reflux.

The most common type of LES dysfunction in GERD results from a disorder of LES opening. Specifically, patients with GERD have too many transient LES relaxations (TLESRs), i.e. episodes when the LES relaxes with the potential for elimination of the pressure gradient between stomach and esophagus and therefore allowing for reflux (Box 1.1). These relaxations seemingly occur in the absence of the normal initiating mechanisms of opening (swallowing, most commonly, although belching and vomiting may cause LES relaxation as well). In fact, they are most commonly seen postprandially, the time when most of us note that reflux occurs. The precise pathophysiology of TLESRs is unclear, although some of the mechanisms may

include distension of the gastric cardia with eating, humoral responses such as those evoked by fat entering the duodenum, the presence of a hiatal hernia, and even central responses through opiate and gamma-aminobutyric acid mechanisms. The basic question of why some people develop these TLESRs and others do not is not known. We do know that TLESRs are the dominant mechanism of reflux in all patients, regardless of whether the patient is upright or lying down, fasting or eating. It seems though that just the presence of TLESRs is not always enough to cause the more severe forms of GERD such as those associated with erosive disease and ulceration of the esophagus or Barrett's esophagus. For these an additional mechanism is most likely needed.

As a result the second, less common but perhaps more damaging predisposition for GERD is a hypotonic LES, i.e. an LES whose basal tone remains chronically low (Box 1.1). When this occurs it makes compounded events such as TLESRs or abdominal strain more capable of eliminating the esophagogastric pressure gradient and thereby causing reflux. As in TLESRs, neither the causative nor ongoing mechanisms of a hyptonic LES are known, although a large hiatal hernia is commonly associated. It is not surprising, therefore, that patients with the more severe forms of GERD, manifested by esophageal mucosal injury and metaplasia, have low LES pressures.

Often LES dysfunction has a supporting cast in its ability to wreak havoc in the esophagus (Box 1.1). This may include

1. poor esophageal motility which results in prolonged esophageal acid exposure because the esophagus cannot return refluxate back into the stomach
2. delayed gastric emptying causing more opportunity for reflux to occur
3. insufficient saliva or salivary components such as epidermal growth factor (without the volume, bicarbonate and healing properties of epidermal growth factor, all con-

---

Box 1.1 Pathophysiology of gastroesophageal reflux disease (GERD)

Defective lower esophageal sphincter (LES) function
   transient LES relaxations (TLESRs)*
   hypotonic LES** (e.g. scleroderma)
   disruption of LES** (e.g. resection, balloon rupture)
Hiatal hernia** (mal-alignment of LES and crural diaphragm)
Poor esophageal clearance**
Decreased salivary protection
   decreased volume (e.g. sicca syndrome)
   deficient production of epidermal growth factor
Poor gastric emptying
Increased intra-abdominal pressure (e.g. straining, obesity, pregnancy)
Duodenogastric reflux (bile)

* Major defect
** Predisposes to severe GERD

tained in saliva, the esophageal mucosa loses a major defense mechanism)
4. poor local defense mechanisms within the esophageal mucosa
5. a mixed gastric refluxate including not only acid but also bile and pepsin which may both cause injury to the esophagus in combination with acid.

Although these factors do not seemingly cause GERD alone, in combination with a defective LES, they contribute strongly to esophageal injury. It is important to recognize this as many of the therapies we use for GERD are in fact aimed more toward these mechanisms rather than primarily at the LES.

Clinical presentation

The cardinal symptom of gastroesophageal reflux is heartburn, classically described as a predictable substernal burning sensation rising up into the chest from the abdomen, usually after meals and relieved by antisecretory therapy or antacids. However, reflux pain can be quite variable and it may be dull or sharp or only a pressure high up in the chest or even low down in the epigastrium. Indeed, distinguishing between pain of esophageal or cardiac origin can be a daunting task; hence ruling out cardiac disease is the most important first step if there is any doubt. We have all seen our share of patients complaining of "heartburn" as a presentation of angina pectoris. Other common symptoms of GERD may also include regurgitation, typically of a sour, bitter material, dysphagia, particularly if a stricture (or, more worrisome, a carcinoma) has developed, and the sensation of food "repeating" (Box 1.2). Occasionally, dysphagia occurs in the absence of a structural lesion when it is due to inflammation alone. Again, these symptoms are non-specific, for example heartburn, regurgitation and food repeating are commonly found in achalasia as well as

> **Box 1.2** Cardinal (classic) symptoms of gastroesophageal reflux disease
>
> Heartburn
> Regurgitation
> Dysphagia
> Other minor symptoms
>   burping
>   bloating
>   early satiety
>   epigastric pain
>   food repeating

GERD. As in most diseases, it is the symptoms, together with the proper precipitating factors, that make the diagnosis possible. Precipitating factors in GERD are many. The most important include high-fat meals (particularly when eaten at night followed by recumbency), caffeine, nicotine and alcohol. Patients may also complain of reflux symptoms after spicy food, tomato sauces, onions, garlic, or acidic juices. The precise pathophysiologic mechanism of reflux symptoms with these specific foods is not well understood nor is it understood why some foods elicit reflux symptoms in some patients but not in others. Although stress is felt to be a significant cause of reflux, in fact the onset of symptoms with stress more likely reflects an increase in esophageal afferent sensation when exposed to acid rather than an absolute increase in reflux per se.

With our ability to diagnose GERD more precisely by using ambulatory pH monitoring (see p. 6), an entirely new group of symptoms attributable to GERD has emerged. These have been termed "extraesophageal" manifestations of GERD because the nature of these symptom/disease complexes is such that they result from the deleterious effect of acid on organs outside the esophagus (Box 1.3). As a result, gastroesophageal reflux can now assume many forms and symptoms ranging from chronic cough and hoarseness to uncontrolled or worsening asthma. Recent studies are pushing the boundaries even further, implicating chronic sinusitis and ear ache as potentially GERD related. Proposed mechanisms include the direct effect of gastric contents on such structures as the vocal cords and bronchi, or reflex mechanisms on these structures through esophageal receptors. One might ask "why not rely upon the coexistence of typical GERD-like symptoms in association with these laryngeal and respiratory-type symptoms to help make the diagnosis?" In fact commonly, and in our experience more likely, typical reflux symptoms are lacking in these patients. As a result, diagnosis of an extra-esophageal presentation of GERD is usually done through objective testing or empiric therapy. One exception to this rule is nasopharyngolaryngoscopy in patients with reflux laryngitis. Changes are seen in approximately 50 per cent of such patients although not all visualized changes are specific for GERD.

Several caveats must be kept in mind when evaluating extraesophageal manifestations of GERD.

1. The documentation of abnormal esophageal acid exposure in these patients represents an association rather than a clearly cause and effect.

2. The cause of these patients' symptoms may be multifactorial (e.g. patients with asthma may have an allergic component as well) where acid reflux is a contributor of unclear magnitude

3. In some situations (e.g. hoarseness secondary to laryngeal injury), physiologic reflux may be implicated as a cause so that objective measures documenting abnormal acid exposure may not be helpful in making a diagnosis. This may be because these extraesophageal structures lack the normal defense mechanisms of the esophagus and thus cannot tolerate similar acid loads. Thus, symptoms such as hoarseness, cough or wheezing may be an important lead for the presence of reflux, but firm conclusions with regard to the precise etiology of these symptoms may be difficult to come by.

Diagnosis

Radiology

For many years, upper gastrointestinal radiography was the cornerstone of the diagnosis of GERD. With the advent of more precise methods such as endoscopy and 24-hour ambulatory esophageal pH monitoring, radiography has lost much of its importance. This is in part because of the general consensus that the very specific signs (esophageal stricture, esophageal ulcer, severe erosive esophagitis) are relatively uncommon whereas the more common signs of GERD such as hiatal hernia or the induction of reflux of barium during the study are very non-specific.

Barium esophagography does have its importance, however, in the assessment of GERD patients in some very specific situations. The first is that any patient with suspected GERD and dysphagia should initially undergo a barium study. This is because with

---

Box 1.3 Extraesophageal manifestations of gastroesophageal reflux disease

Non-cardiac chest pain
ENT symptoms
 chronic hoarseness
 voice strain and vocal cord granulomas
 posterior laryngitis
 subglottic stenosis
 globus sensation
 laryngeal cancer in non-smokers
 others (sinusitis, otalgia and otitis media, dental enamel loss)
Bronchopulmonary symptoms
 adult onset asthma
 chronic cough with normal chest X-ray
 others (idiopathic pulmonary fibrosis, sleep apnea)

strong suspicion of stricture and/or carcinoma, it is preferable to be prepared at the time of planned endoscopy to deal with these possibilities. For example, in the presence of a long reflux-induced stricture, one will be prepared for dilation and will know the type of dilator to be used and whether the procedure should be performed under fluoroscopy. In contrast, for a patient with suspected adenocarcinoma-complicating GERD, one might plan endoscopic ultrasound at the same time. Barium studies are also helpful preoperatively when planning for surgical fundoplication. For example, patients with large hiatal hernias may require a chest approach or may need an esophageal-lengthening procedure in addition to the usual wrap. This must be known prior to surgery. Finally, barium studies of the esophagus may also be helpful in differentiating GERD from other diseases that may mimic the symptoms of GERD such as achalasia or a Zenker's diverticulum (much more easily diagnosed on esophagram than endoscopy). Thus, barium contrast study of the esophagus may not be the best first line tool for the diagnosis of GERD, but it still has some important roles in its management.

Endoscopy

Endoscopic visualization of the esophagus is the first-line objective test in the diagnosis of GERD. Although only a minority (perhaps 20 per cent) of patients will have gross esophagitis, the finding of erosive reflux disease (ERD) as opposed to non-erosive reflux disease (NERD) has tremendous implications with regard to prognosis and therapy. Although good prospective data are lacking, we know that if an adult patient has NERD at the time of initial endoscopy, it is uncommon for ERD to develop at a future time. In other words, it appears that the extent of esophageal injury an adult will sustain as a result of GERD is determined fairly early on in adulthood and remains stable. Consequently, the primary intent of therapy is for symptom control rather than prevention of more serious disease. On the other hand, the finding of ERD predicts lifelong risk of recurrent erosive disease if therapy were to be stopped or if it is suboptimal. Moreover, the finding of Barrett's epithelium is considered a manifestation of marked esophageal injury secondary to acid reflux, which requires an aggressive pharmacologic approach. Thus, the finding of erosive esophagitis or Barrett's esophagus on endoscopy demands lifelong intensive anti-reflux therapy.

One of the dilemmas in endoscopic evaluation of reflux disease has been determining which histologic or endoscopic changes really constitute significant injury. For years pathologists have relied on findings such as eosinophils and neutrophils in the squamous mucosa as diagnostic of reflux even in the face of a normal endoscopic appearance. Similarly, endoscopists may describe "mild" esophagitis given by hyperemia of the distal esophageal mucosa. The current approach, however, is to consider erosive esophagitis in a similar way to pregnancy — either it's there or it isn't. Along this vein a recent classification for ERD has been proposed termed the Los Angeles Classification Scale. In this scale esophagitis is divided into four categories, A to D, in order of severity. Besides attempting to standardize the way we all rate esophagitis, this classification also starts off with at least one or more grossly visible mucosal breaks up to 5 mm in length (grade A). As a result, it attempts to avoid the overcall of gross esophageal injury noted in the past and thereby avoid overzealous therapy in those patients for whom symptom control rather than mucosal injury is the main issue. In our experience, histologic assessment adds little to the endoscopic diagnosis of GERD and it is unnecessary unless Barrett's esophagus is suspected or documented in which case it is mandatory for confirmation and for risk stratification depending on the presence or absence of dysplasia.

Ambulatory pH monitoring

Twenty-four hour ambulatory esophageal pH monitoring is presently the gold standard for diagnosing gastroesophageal reflux. It does so by placement of a nasogastric catheter containing usually two to three pH probes that are positioned at standardized points relative to the lower esophageal sphincter. Specifically, pH probes are located in the gastric body, 5 cm above the proximal border of the LES, and a third probe may be placed 20 cm proximal to the LES. Through this placement, acid exposure is measured in the stomach, distal and proximal esophagus. In essence, then, this test defines the presence of acid reflux. Note, however, that pH is not a direct measure of acid volume and it also cannot determine the presence of non-acid reflux (e.g. food). Furthermore, false-negative tests can occur for a variety of reasons. First, since TLESRs are normal phenomena, a certain degree of esophageal acid exposure is physiologic (up to 4.2 per cent at 5 cm above the LES in our laboratory). Second, many patients may limit their normal activities while the probe is in place because of discomfort or embarrassment. Third, technical issues, perhaps due to mucus covering the tip of the catheter or temporary embedding of the probe in the esophageal wall, may also lead to false-negative results.

Inherent in its name is the fact that this test is completely ambulatory. Patients routinely have the catheter placed while they are in the hospital or laboratory. The patients are then able to leave and return the next day to have the catheter removed, and data are downloaded from a data recorder attached to the catheter worn on the trouser belt for the duration of the study. Although not always possible, patients are encouraged to carry on their normal activities as best as possible with the catheter in place. Indeed, patients are encouraged to pursue activities which normally cause reflux. This in turn points out another advantage of this test over other tests for reflux, and that is the chance to correlate the patient's symptoms with the occurrence of reflux episodes. It is generally believed that a symptom index of greater than 50 per cent (i.e. when more than 50 per cent of symptom episodes are associated with periods of acid exposure in the distal esophagus) has a high predictive value for the presence of GERD.

As valuable as ambulatory pH monitoring is in the diagnosis of GERD, it is still evolving in terms of its indications. There are several reasons why it is clearly not needed for primary diagnosis in a patient with the onset of classic GERD symptoms. First, as discussed above (see p. 5), endoscopy alone provides valuable information as a guide to treatment. Second, with proton pump inhibitors as effective as they are, patients are often started on empiric therapy rather than be subjected to this test. Third, the availability of pH monitoring is variable, more commonly used at tertiary referral centres than in community practices because of the need for a well-trained technician to perform the test and physicians knowledgable in the area for interpretation. As a result, at present pH monitoring is generally reserved for some of the following indications:

1. documentation of acid reflux in the patient refractory to medical therapy
2. documentation of acid reflux in a patient considering surgical fundoplication
3. to demonstrate objective proof of adequate control of acid reflux in a patient with high-grade erosive esophagitis or Barrett's where symptoms often underestimate acid exposure
4. documentation of the presence of acid reflux in patients with extraesophageal or atypical manifestations of GERD, where typical symptoms of acid reflux are often lacking.

An example of an ambulatory pH study is given in Figure 1.1.

Proton pump inhibitor test

Because of the potency of proton pump inhibitors, particularly in twice daily dosing, some authors have advocated a response to therapy with these agents as a test for GERD in and of itself. Indeed, the results of studies comparing symptom response to ambulatory pH monitoring are surprisingly similar in accuracy. In practice, this strategy is probably followed quite commonly, accounting for the very high use of proton pump inhibitors in this country. Two strong caveats must be kept in mind in using this "test", however. First, a response to a proton pump inhibitor does not define a pathologic diagnosis. Thus, whether a patient has underlying Barrett's esophagus or peptic esophagitis is unknown at the start of therapy. We therefore advocate a once-in-a-lifetime endoscopy in all proton pump inhibitor dependent patients to exclude the presence of Barrett's esophagus which modifies management. Furthermore, patients with ERD may now be masked by empiric therapy, making a future guide to therapy not available if patients are endoscoped months after empiric treatment has begun. Finally, this method of diagnosis is probably not as useful in patients with extraesophageal manifestations of GERD. In general, empiric proton pump inhibitor trials in such patients need to be at high doses for prolonged periods.

Other studies

Esophageal manometry has only a minor role to play in the diagnostic work-up of patients with GERD. This procedure is able to identify some of the secondary features of the disease such as a low, resting, LES pressure or ineffective motility. However, as mentioned previously, these features only tend to be of relevance when they occur together with more important defining pathophysiologic criteria such as frequent TLESRs (which manometry cannot identify readily; this requires specialized ambulatory equipment which is still considered experimental) or hiatal hernias (which are better identified endoscopically or radiographically). Manometry does have utility in the preoperative work-up of patients undergoing fundoplication operations (see p. 12) or to define the precise level at which to place 24-hour ambulatory esophageal probes.

Recently there has been a significant interest displayed in a new technique which measures esophageal impedance. Although this technique is still firmly in the research realm, it may become a valuable tool for identifying the presence of non-acid refluxate.

Table 1.1 lists the major diagnostic approaches in patients suspected of having GERD.

Therapy

Types of treatment

Before giving specific recommendations for the treatment of GERD patients, the available types of treatments must first be defined. These include 1) lifestyle changes, 2) antacids, 3) histamine H_2-receptor antagonists, 4) proton pump inhibitors, 5) surgical fundoplication, and 6) new endoscopic treatments (Table 1.2). The decision on which approaches are needed for which patients depends largely on the severity of their disease. Each of these therapies has its place in treatment, some in combination with others, some at one stage of the disease, some at other stages. Each will be discussed individually. At the present time, prokinetic agents are no longer considered standard therapy for GERD and medications that reduce the frequency of TLESRs such as

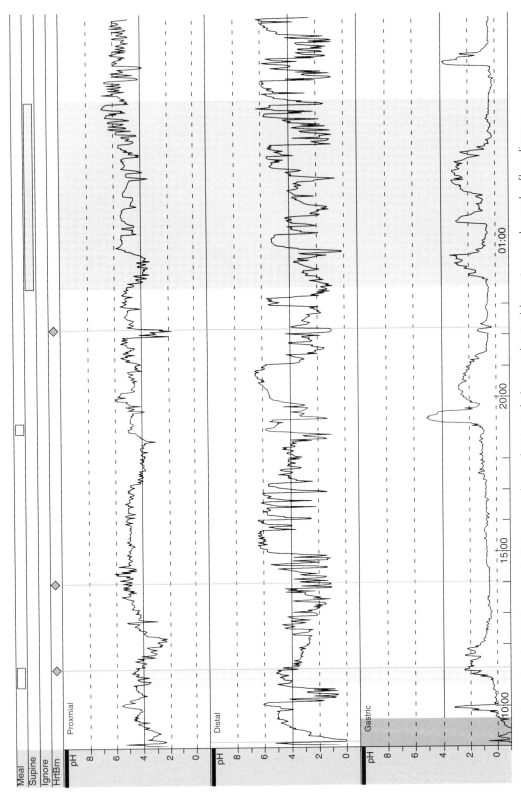

Figure 1.1 Example of a 24-hour ambulatory esophageal pH study in a patient with gastroesophageal reflux disease: hours, *y* axis is pH. Three panels from top to bottom represent tracings of proximal esophageal acid exposur esophageal sphincter (LES)), distal esophageal acid exposure (5 cm above the LES) and gastric-acid exposure (10 Symptoms, meal timing, and patient position are given in the top legend. In the middle panel note the frequent episodes of gastroesophageal reflux when esophageal pH dips below 4. Also note the occurrence of heartburn symptoms (vertical lines) showin excellent correlation with acid reflux events.

Table 1.1 Diagnostic tests for gastroesophageal reflux disease

Test	Advantages	Disadvantages	Comments
Endoscopy	establishes severity diagnoses Barrett's	expensive often normal	Most useful in the presence of effective symptom control.
Barium X-ray	defines anatomy in patients with dysphagia	often normal or non-specific	Useful to exclude mimickers or to plan surgery.
Ambulatory esophageal pHmetry	quantifies reflux monitors efficacy of therapy permits calculation of symptom index	false negatives occur expensive	Current gold standard. May be done on or off therapy.
Oral proton pump inhibitor test	diagnostic and therapeutic cheap no expertise required	may mask underlying disease precludes stratification of disease severity less accurate for extraesophageal disease	Therapy b.i.d. for 1 week in esophageal or non-cardiac chest-pain patients. Longer trials for extraesophageal disease patients. Responders still need an endoscopy to exclude Barrett's.
Esophageal manometry	identifies low LES pressures (patients at risk for severe disease)	limited application	Major use is preoperative or to aid in pH probe placement.
Esophageal impedance	identifies non-acid reflux	clinical utility not clear	Still experimental.

LES lower esophageal sphincter

opioid receptor antagonists are still under study but are not yet ready for routine use.

Lifestyle changes

Recommendations for lifestyle change for GERD are numerous. Some have a good scientific basis while others are more anecdotal. The most important recommendation is to avoid large-volume high-fat diets, particularly before bedtime (Box 1.4). Fats exacerbate reflux by several mechanisms. First, they increase the number of TLESRs. Second, they lower LES tone. Third, they increase esophageal sensitivity to acid. Fourth, they delay gastric emptying, which may also contribute to reflux. Our feeling is that even patients on proton pump inhibitors should avoid night-time, high-volume, high-fat meals to prevent non-acid reflux.

After that, the data are a little less strong for avoiding other agents. Caffeine, alcohol, mints and chocolate have all been shown to lower LES pressure, and some have been shown to increase acid exposure. In the patient who is not on any medical treatment where one or more of these agents clearly invokes symptoms, it is best to avoid them. It

Table 1.2 Therapeutic approaches in gastroesophageal reflux disease (GERD)

Therapeutic approach	Comments
Lifestyle modifications	Advisable in all patients.
	Of limited use in isolation.
Over the counter therapies (antacids and half-strength H₂RAs)	Useful for mild, intermittent GERD.
	Combination agents now available.
Prescription H₂RAs	Less effective than proton pump inhibitors.
Proton pump inhibitors.	First-line therapy.
	Once daily treatment effective in about 85% of esophageal patients.
Fundoplication	Laparoscopic approaches are likely to be as effective as open surgery.
	Efficacy may be as short as 10 years.
	Requires careful preoperative gastrointestinal evaluation.
	Most successful in patients who respond to proton pump inhibitors.
Newer therapies (radiofrequency ablation, lower esophageal sphincter injection, sewing machine)	Only non-erosive reflux disease patients without hiatal hernias.
	Still experimental.

Box 1.4 Lifestyle modifications for gastroesophageal reflux disease (GERD)

Avoid large volume meals just before bed
Avoid meals with high fat content
Avoid other foods that may precipitate or exacerbate GER
  caffeine
  alcohol
  mints
  chocolate
  acidic foods (tomatoes, nuts, citrus fruits)
Avoid tobacco products
Avoid eating before exercise
Weight loss
Stress reduction
Elevate head of bed 6 inches
Sleep on left side rather than right
Avoid tight-fitting clothes

Others have discussed the refluxogenic nature of foods such as tomato products, citrus juices, nuts, etc. These foods do not have to be assiduously avoided unless they clearly cause symptoms. In the presence of pharmacologic therapy, these foods are much better tolerated.

Cigarette smoking should, of course, be avoided in general, but from an esophageal point of view, it does lower LES pressure and may interfere with local defense mechanisms against the damage of acid.

Weight loss should be encouraged in overweight individuals because of general health concerns and also because it may reduce intra-abdominal pressure. Avoidance of tight-fitting clothes may also be beneficial.

Exercise after heavy meals should be avoided because of the increase in abdominal pressure that occurs with exercise. In patients with known low LES pressure, this may be enough to overcome sphincter competence. The role of stress in GERD is unclear. It most likely increases symptoms because of an augmenta-

is unlikely that these agents cause enough acid exposure to injure the esophageal epithelium but this has not been well studied.

tion of esophageal afferent sensation rather than an induction of reflux. In other words, it probably worsens the symptoms but not the reflux. Stress reduction methods will help symptoms only to a limited extent.

Finally, the role of body position is unclear. Reflux patients display different patterns of reflux, some upright, some supine and some with both. It is generally thought that the nocturnal, supine reflux is the most injurious. We have already suggested remaining upright after meals. Other methods such as raising the head of the bed may also help supine refluxers. More recent data suggest that lying prone or on the left side causes less reflux than lying on the right side or in the supine position. It is certainly hard to control body position during sleep but starting in a more advantageous position may be of help.

Antacids and histamine H_2-receptor antagonists

Over-the-counter type therapies for GERD, such as antacids and half-prescription-strength histamine H_2-receptor antagonists, are useful for occasional (as needed) therapy. Antacids are limited by a relatively short duration of action (1 to 3 hours generally) leading to inconvenience and the potential for side effects (e.g. diarrhea or constipation from magnesium- or aluminum-containing antacids respectively) from the need to take multiple doses throughout the day. Histamine H_2-receptor antagonists have a longer duration of action than antacids and seem preferable. They are also more efficacious when taken prophylactically. One criticism of on-demand histamine H_2-receptor antagonists has been the slow onset of action due to the requirement for systemic absorption from the gut. This has recently been overcome to a large extent by formulations that dissolve on the tongue. In addition, combination antacid plus histamine H_2-receptor antagonist medication have recently been marketed as an over-the-counter formulation. Full-prescrip-

tion-strength histamine H_2-receptor antagonist therapy is useful for only the milder forms of GERD and even double-dose therapy is not as effective as proton pump inhibitor therapy for patients with more severe forms of GERD.

Proton pump inhibitors

These medications have become the cornerstone of therapy because of their potent ability to inhibit gastric-acid secretion. This is achieved by pharmacologic inhibition of the H^+–K^+ adenosine triphosphatase in the parietal cell secretory canaliculus, the final common pathway of acid secretion. As a result, these drugs avoid some of the pitfalls of histamine H_2-receptor antagonists, such as tachyphylaxis at the receptor level (proton pump inhibitors bind an ionic pump, not a receptor) and suboptimal control of acid secretion because of undertreatment. A single dose of omeprazole is enough to keep the gastric pH above 4 for more than 50 per cent of the day on average. In doses of 20 mg twice daily, pH above 4 approaches 70 per cent of the day. Furthermore, these medications are safe in both short- and long-term studies. Specifically, some of the early fears that surrounded the chronic use of proton pump inhibitors such as the development of enterochromaffin-like cell carcinoid tumors of the stomach, vitamin B_{12} deficiency and predisposition to bacterial overgrowth have not turned out to be clinically significant risks in up to 13 years of documented continuous use. It should not be surprising then that this class of drug has become the most commonly prescribed medication in the world. One ongoing controversy is whether the newer generation proton pump inhibitors (i.e. rabeprazole, esomeprazole or pantoprazole) are superior to the first generation proton pump inhibitors (i.e. omeprazole or lansoprazole). There may be subtle differences in duration of acid inhibition but in regular clinical practice they are all excellent agents. Once daily therapy is effective in approximately 85 per cent of all patients with typical heartburn. One pitfall of proton pump inhibitors that the newer generation drugs have tried to address is the control of nocturnal reflux. Although some may achieve better control than others, there is still a significant prevalence of a recently recognized phenomenon termed "nocturnal acid breakthrough". The clinical significance of this phenomenon is still being debated and it may purely be a manifestation of the normal diurnal variation of gastric-acid production. No clinical studies have yet demonstrated a convincing relationship between nocturnal acid breakthrough (defined as a sustained drop in gastric pH below 4 during the early morning hours) and poor symptom control in reflux patients on proton pump inhibitor therapy. Finally, one important aspect regarding the use of proton pump inhibitors is the need for administration 30 to 60 minutes before a meal. Patients commonly make the mistake of taking proton pump inhibitors either in the morning and then skipping breakfast, or right before bedtime. This subtle recommendation may make a huge difference in some patients because proton pump inhibitors are pro-drugs that become activated in the acidic milieu of the secretory canaliculus following activation of proton pumps by a preceding meal.

Fundoplication

Surgical fundoplication has been in use for several decades with proven long-term efficacy. Indeed, 10- and 20-year studies from institutions which have surgical expertise in esophageal disease demonstrate up to 90 per cent continued success. Although a recent study has challenged the success rate of fundoplication, it still remains an excellent option in the management of GERD.

Several types of fundoplication may be performed, usually varying by the extent of the wrap. Specifically, the priniciple of the fundoplication is a wrapping of the proximal stomach around the distal esophagus and lower esophageal sphincter. Although it was originally thought that this operation works by increasing tonic pressure in the area of the sphincter, it may also work by inhibition of TLESRs or by recreating the angle of Hiss and returning the hiatal hernia sac to the abdominal cavity. The type of wrap is defined by how much of the stomach is pulled around the esophagus. For example, in the standard Nissen fundoplication, portions of the stomach are pulled all the way around making a 360-degree wrap. Similarly, surgeons may create 270- and 180-degree wraps. As one might expect, the tighter the wrap the better the control of reflux. In patients with extremely poor esophageal peristalsis, where creation of a new high-pressure zone in the distal esophagus may cause dysphagia, lesser degree wraps are used.

With the ability to perform fundoplications laparoscopically, the surgical approach to reflux has become a much more attractive form of therapy recently. Five-year studies show equal efficacy to the open approach with the attending advantages of much shorter hospital stay and less postoperative pain. It is important to remember though that the other aspects of postoperative recovery are otherwise the same. Patients commonly have dysphagia for the first month and routinely follow a restrictive liquid and soft diet during that time. Most surgeons recommend at least 2 weeks before returning to work. Patients may have prolonged early satiety, flatulence and "gas bloat syndrome" (inability to belch with subsequent air retention in the stomach). There is less than a 1 per cent mortality but, rarely, patients have have inadvertant splenic trauma or vagus nerve damage. Long-term complications include herniation and breakdown of the wrap.

One of the most important aspects of deciding upon fundoplication is the choice of the surgeon. Most experts in the field estimate a learning curve of at least 100 operations before a surgeon feels comfortable with all parts of the procedure. Patients also have to be very carefully evaluated prior to fundoplication with manometry, barium and endoscopic studies, and most likely pH monitoring in the absence of gross erosive esophagitis or Barrett's esophagus. In our experience, the greatest failures of fundoplication are those patients who have not been carefully evaluated preoperatively. We feel strongly that fundoplication works best for those patients with documented reflux who have responded to proton pump inhibitor therapy.

Newer therapies

Several recent experimental therapies have been applied to GERD. These include an endoscopic suturing device which in essence creates a gastroplasty, a transoral catheter unit that delivers radiofrequency to the LES with the idea of fibrosing the area and inhibiting TLESRs, endoscopic injection of the LES with substances that also may fibrose or expand the area, and others. Thus far, these experimental approaches have been limited to patients with NERD and no hiatal hernias who do not want to take life-long proton pump inhibitor therapy, although these are precisely the patients who do best with low-dose treatment. Preliminary results from the first two types of therapy have been published and do show some efficacy with regard to symptoms, but ambulatory esophageal pH data suggest much of the effect may be due to visceral sensory inhibition rather than prevention of esophageal acid exposure. No follow-up longer than 1 year has been obtained, and they have only been tested in relatively small numbers of motivated patients so general applicability at this time is unclear. We do not advocate these procedures routinely for use in reflux disease at this time but further study and refinements of these techniques may dramatically change the way we treat GERD patients in the future.

Specific treatment recommendations

Decisions regarding the treatment of GERD are aimed at three different types of patients:
- those with erosive reflux disease
- those with non-erosive reflux disease
- those with extraesophageal manifestations of reflux disease.

This having been said, since we still believe in empiric, diagnostic and treatment trials in patients without significant risk for serious pathology (i.e. young patients with new onset of symptoms in the absence of weight loss, dysphagia, anemia or bleeding), the distinction between erosive and non-erosive disease may not be readily apparent and, in fact, once rendered asymptomatic the upper endoscopy can often be deferred until proton pump inhibitor dependence is identified. We believe that such patients should be treated as if they had erosive disease since almost all patients respond to proton pump inhibitors.

Patients with erosive reflux disease are generally easy to manage. They need life-long therapy with proton pump inhibitors or they need a fundoplication. The reason for this approach is as follows. For patients with erosive disease, the healing rate, when treated with anything less than a proton pump inhibitor or surgery, is less than 40 per cent. The relapse rate once healed is greater than 80 per cent. With these types of compelling data, it is easy to understand the nature of this firm recommendation. Intuitively, this makes sense as the amount of acid reflux necessary to cause severe esophageal damage is more than a histamine H_2-receptor antagonist is capable of controlling pharmacologically. Given this recommendation, the only confusing aspect to this dictum is the dose of proton pump inhibitor to be used. On once daily omeprazole, the healing rate of high-grade esophagitis is approximately 70 to 90 per cent. As a result, many esophagologists advocate twice daily use of a proton pump inhibitor, once before breakfast and once before dinner. As mentioned previously, one of the hopes of the newer proton pump inhibitors is the ability to use once daily dosing. Efficacy may approach 90 per cent in some of these studies. It really comes down to how "guaranteed" one wants to be of controlling the reflux, remembering also that it is primarily the night-time reflux that causes the most injury. At this point we use twice daily therapy liberally and we aim for an absolutely symptom-free patient. However, because freedom from symptoms does not always assure the absence of erosive disease, if once daily use is to be tried in erosive-disease patients, then consideration should be given to performing an ambulatory pH study on medication to prove adequate control, or a repeat endoscopy 6 to 12 months later can be done to ensure maintenance of healing. Similar strategies may be taken after the performance of a fundoplication. Although excellent at healing and maintaining esophagitis, it is not 100 per cent successful and long-term monitoring of efficacy may be worthwhile as well. It must be stressed that such an aggressive approach may not be embraced by all experts in the field.

Patients with NERD are a little more complicated with regard to the endpoint of treatment. The two possible endpoints of treatment are prevention of future injury (esophagitis, Barrett's) and control of symptoms. There are no good prospective data on what the risk is of developing more severe forms of esophageal disease in those patients who present with reflux symptoms and a normal-appearing esophagus. As mentioned previously, we think the risk is small and at this time advocate treatment for the purpose of symptom control only. It is important to keep in mind, however, that many if not most patients who are sent for endoscopy have been treated already, so a normal-appearing esophagus may not guarantee little risk of

future esophageal injury. In these patients, a pH study while off medications to objectively assess the magnitude of acid reflux may be helpful. Assuming that for most of these patients the endpoint will be symptom control, then the use of a specific drug or surgery depends on the frequency and severity of symptoms. For patients with sporadic and/or predictable symptoms after identifiable precipitating factors have been managed by lifestyle modification, histamine H_2-receptor antagonists may be very effective. In general clinical gastroenterological practice this turns out to be a minority of patients. For patients with either daily or several times per week symptoms, proton pump inhibitors are the more likely drugs of choice. Frequency and strength of dosage can be titrated to symptom control. Recent studies have brought out the concept of "step-down" therapy; that is after a course of proton pump inhibitors, trying to then use histamine H_2-receptor antagonists for maintenance therapy. Although these studies have documented reasonable success with this strategy, in our experience, most patients with true GERD will request to be maintained on proton pump inhibitors because of their superior efficacy in controlling symptoms. Fundoplication is an option in these patients as well, especially in those with ambulatory pH-proven disease who can not or will not take maintenance therapy. Although one might think of erosive disease and Barrett's as the main indication for fundoplication, the majority of patients undergoing surgery have NERD. There are no clear recommendations on which patients should undergo fundoplication other than those proven refractory to proton pump inhibitors (an extremely rare occurrence in compliant patients). Some have advocated that younger patients who may face life-long therapy with GERD should consider fundoplication, but less than 20-year follow-up on this procedure, as well as some recent studies examining the use of reflux medication in

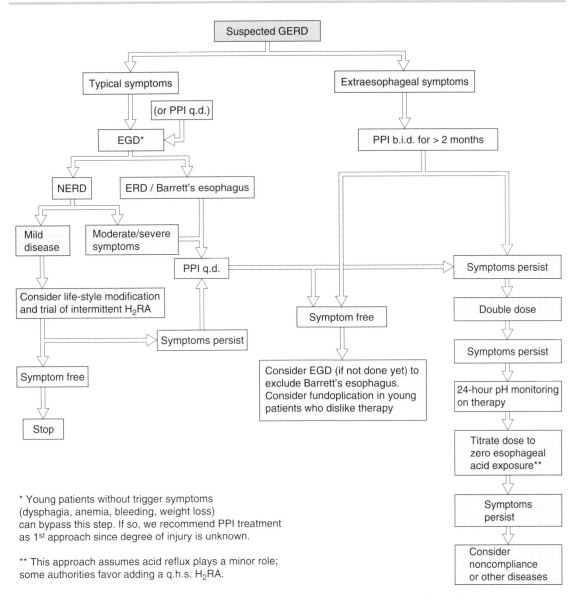

Figure 1.2 An algorithmic approach to gastroesophageal reflux disease (GERD). PPI proton pump inhibitors; EGD upper endoscopy; ERD erosive reflux disease; NERD non-erosive reflux disease; H₂RA histamine H₂-receptor antagonist.

patients post-fundoplication, make it quite clear that surgery is by no means a guarantee of obviating the need for future medication. At this point we offer healthy, good-surgical-risk patients both medical and surgical options although we are biased toward continued medical therapy.

Patients with atypical manifestations of GERD are probably the most challenging subset of patients with GERD for reasons discussed previously. Because of these problems, these patients are treated very aggressively pharmacologically. Indeed, we try to push them almost toward achlorhydria with virtually zero esophageal acid exposure so as to best evaluate what role GERD has in the generation of their symptoms. We use high-dose, twice daily, proton pump inhibitor therapy in all patients. If symptoms persist, then ambulatory pH monitoring on therapy should be considered. The potential role of an additional night-time histamine H_2-recptor antagonist for nocturnal acid breakthrough is controversial. It should be noted that this approach does not eliminate the possibility of "non-acid" reflux persisting. Surgery should preferably be used only in those patients with proven reflux, particularly those with a good response to medical therapy and other objective data showing that reflux is occurring. Occasionally, one sees a patient so desperate, for example a severe steroid dependent, commonly hospitalized, asthmatic patient where fundoplication is performed in the hope that it will help, but this is one of the more difficult decisions to make and should only be made by a team of esophagologists, pulmonologists and an esophageal surgeon. Finally, one other caveat must be kept in mind regarding treatment. Unlike more typical manifestations of GERD, the extreme sensitivity of extraesophageal structures to acid dictates an empiric trial of therapy lasting for up to 6 months before a response to therapy may be considered a failure. Figure 1.2 illustrates an algorithmic approach to erosive, non-erosive and extraesophageal reflux disease.

Further reading

Cameron AJ, Lagergren J, Henriksson C, *et al.* Gastroesophageal reflux disease in monozygotic twins. *Gastroenterology* 2002; 122: 55–59.

Eubanks TR, Omelanczuk E, Maronian N, *et al.* Pharyngeal pH monitoring in 222 patients with suspected laryngeal reflux. *J Gastrointest Surg* 2001; 5: 183–191.

Fass R, Fennerty MB, Ofman JJ, *et al.* The clinical and economic value of a short course of omeprazole in patients with noncardiac chest pain. *Gastroenterology* 1998; 115: 42–49.

Inadomi JM, Jamal R, Murata G, *et al.* Step-down management of gastroesophageal reflux disease. *Gastroenterology* 2001; 121: 1095–1100.

Klinkenberg-Knol EC, Nelis F, Dent J, *et al.* Long-term omeprazole treatment in resistant gastroesophageal reflux disease: efficacy, safety, and influence on gastric mucosa. *Gastroenterology* 2000; 118: 661–669.

Mittal RK. Transient lower esophageal sphincter relaxation. *Gastroenterology* 1995; 109: 601–612.

Peghini PL, Katz PO, Castell DO. Ranitadine controls nocturnal gastric acid breakthrough on omeprazole: a controlled study in normal subjects. *Gastroenterology* 1998; 115: 1335–1339.

Spechler SJ, Lee E, Ahnen D, *et al.* Long-term outcome of medical and surgical therapies for gastroesophageal reflux disease. *JAMA* 2001; 285: 2331–2337.

Vigneri S, Termini R, Leandro G, *et al.* A comparison of five maintenance therapies for reflux esophagitis. *N Engl J Med* 1995; 333: 1106–1110.

Chapter 2

Other Causes of Esophagitis

John C. Sun and David A. Katzka

Introduction

When most clinicians consider esophagitis, they overwhelmingly think of reflux-induced injury. In fact, many etiologies of non–reflux esophagitis exist, and most can be broken down into a few groups (Box 2.1). This chapter will explore the causes of non–reflux esophagitis, and will discuss their clinical manifestations, diagnosis, and treatment.

Infectious esophagitis

Background

The emergence of human immunodeficiency virus (HIV) and acquired immunodeficiency syndrome (AIDS), and the development

---

Box 2.1 Non-reflux causes of esophagitis

Infectious causes
Candida spp.
herpes simplex virus
cytomegalovirus
mycobacteria
other fungi
  histoplasmosis
  aspergillosis
bacteria
  Staphyloccus spp.
  Streptococcus spp.

Pill-induced causes
non-steroidal anti-inflammatory drugs
antibiotics
cardiac medications
alendronate

Corrosive causes
acids
alkalis

Radiation-induced causes
acute
chronic

---

of immunosuppressive therapy for transplantation and other diseases have increased the number of cases and causes of infectious esophagitis. Physicians should maintain a high index of suspicion for an infectious etiology in patients presenting with odynophagia. Rapid diagnosis of the etiologic agent, based upon consistent signs and symptoms, and gross and histologic evidence, is important because effective treatment exists for infectious esophagitis.

This section will deal with the common causes of infectious esophagitis, and address them with respect to both immunocompetent as well as immunocompromised hosts. Esophagitis in patients with AIDS deserves special consideration and will be discussed in detail.

Epidemiology and risk factors

With perhaps the exception of esophagitis due to herpes simplex virus (HSV), infectious esophagitis is unusual in a truly immunocompetent host; more commonly, patients have some degree of compromise of their cell-mediated or humoral immunity (Table 2.1).

"Immunocompetent" hosts that develop infectious esophagitis usually possess local or systemic factors that predispose to infection. Examples of such predisposing causes include local factors such as esophageal motility disorders, strictures, diverticula, systemic sclerosis, achalasia, myositis, and Chagas' disease. These disorders cause esophageal stasis leading to increased risk of infection. Additionally, certain systemic conditions may also increase host susceptibility to esophageal infection. Diabetes mellitus, malnutrition, and substance or alcohol abuse all lead to a functional impairment of the immune system.

Immunodeficiency caused by HIV, use of immunosuppressive medications for autoimmune diseases or transplantation, and bone-marrow transplantation all predispose to infectious esophagitis. In post-transplantation patients, bacterial and fungal infections usually occur during the first months as a result of compromised granulocyte function. Viral infection may occur early or later due to neutropenia and impaired T-cell function. In HIV patients, esophageal infections tend to occur when CD4 counts fall below 200 per mm^3.

Candida esophagitis

Epidemiology

Candida is the most common cause of infectious esophagitis overall, and the most common cause of infectious esophagitis in patients with AIDS, accounting for more than 50% of esophageal infections in this popula-

Table 2.1 Risk factors for infectious esophagitis	
Local factors	
Esophageal motility disorders: achalasia systemic sclerosis Chagas' disease Esophageal diverticula Strictures	Interferes with esophageal emptying and promotes esophageal stasis.
Local chemo- or radiation therapy	Disrupts mucosal barrier.
Systemic factors	
Diabetes mellitus	Impairs granulocyte function.
Malnutrition	Impairs immune function.
Alcohol or illicit substance abuse Older age Malignancies	
Glucocorticoid use or excess	Interferes with granulocyte and neutrophil function.
Immunocompromised state	
Post-transplantation	Immunosuppressive medications compromise host immune defenses.
HIV	Impairs cellular immunity, and affects humoral immunity secondarily.

tion. Although *Candida albicans* is the most prevalent species, infections with *C. tropicalis*, *C. glabrata* and *C. parapsilosis* may also occur. Candida esophagitis may represent the sole cause of esophagitis in AIDS patients, or may exist with other infectious agents, such as cytomegalovirus. Candida esophagitis is summarized in Box 2.2.

Risk factors

Candida species are part of normal oral flora, and their growth is usually kept in check by other native flora. Host cellular immunity serves to limit candidal growth, and neutrophil defense serves to prevent systemic disease. When alterations occur in the oral flora, or when host immune function is compromised, candida infection may occur.

Risk factors for candida infection include the following.

1. Antibiotic use which alters the normal oral flora allowing for candida overgrowth.
2. Immunosuppressive medications such as glucocorticoids or cytotoxic agents, which compromise immune function, particularly cell-mediated immunity.
3. Host factors such as diabetes mellitus, advanced age, and malnutrition, which may impair immune defenses.
4. Local factors, such as
   - esophageal dysmotility (due to achalasia, systemic sclerosis, etc.)
   - loss of gastric-acid production (from atrophic gastritis or use of acid-blocking medications), which causes alterations in normal physiologic defenses to esophageal infection
   - esophageal intramural pseudodiverticulosis (associated with positive candidal cultures in 48% of cases, and with candidal invasion of tissue in 24% of cases).

Box 2.2 Candida esophagitis

Epidemiology
Most common cause of infectious esophagitis overall.
Increased risk in AIDS patients with a CD4 count less than 200 per mm^3.

Risk factors
Antibiotic use (alters normal oral flora).
Esophageal stasis or dysmotility due to achalasia, systemic sclerosis, etc.
Decreased gastric acid production.
Esophageal intramural pseudodiverticulosis
Compromised host immune system:
   diabetes mellitus, older age, malnutrition, alcohol or drug abuse
   HIV, use of immunosuppressive medications, chronic mucocutaneous candidiasis.

Symptoms and signs
Odynophagia, dysphagia, substernal chest pain.
Decreased oral intake, dehydration, malnutrition.
In AIDS patients, oral thrush and symptoms consistent with esophagitis have a high predictive value for candida esophagitis.

Diagnosis
Upper endoscopy with biopsy and brushings is optimal test:
   grossly, may see white plaques
   send for potassium hydroxide preparation, histologic examination.

Therapy
Fluconazole loading dose of 200 mg p.o. on day 1, then 100 mg p.o. daily for 14 days.
Itraconazole solution 200 mg p.o. daily for 14 days is alternate therapy for fluconazole-resistant cases.
Amphotericin B 0.5 mg/kg daily for 7 days is used in patients not tolerating oral medications, or for azole-resistant cases.

5. Genetic or acquired immune deficiencies such as HIV infection or chronic mucocutaneous candidiasis, which decrease cellular immunity.

Clinical manifestations

Patients with candida esophagitis classically present with odynophagia, dysphagia, and substernal chest pain. The severity of symptoms may range from mild swallowing difficulty to intense pain that prevents swallowing leading to dehydration and malnutrition. Patients who present with particularly severe pain should be worked up for alternate or co-existing diagnoses.

Physical examination of patients with AIDS may reveal oral candidiasis or thrush. Two-thirds of AIDS patients with oral candidiasis and symptoms of esophagitis have candida esophagitis. In patients with chronic mucocutaneous candidiasis (part of the polyglandular autoimmune syndrome type I), fungal infections of other mucosal surfaces, hair, skin, and nails may be present. These patients may also have evidence of primary adrenal insufficiency, such as hyperpigmentation or hypotension.

Diagnosis

Barium esophagram may reveal multiple plaque-like lesions that occur in a linear or confluent fashion. Other findings that may be present include cobblestoning, nodules, fungal balls, strictures, ulcers, masses, or fistulas within the pulmonary tree. A normal esophagram does not exclude candida esophagitis. In addition, the presence of a large ulcer should suggest an alternate diagnosis.

Blind cytology via an oral or nasal approach with brush or balloon technique in AIDS patients has been shown to be sensitive for diagnosis of candida esophagitis, but not for HSV or CMV esophagitis, which may co-exist. Therefore, blind cytology is not an optimal test to determine all possible etiologies of esophagitis in a patient with AIDS.

Upper endoscopy with brush and biopsy has the highest sensitivity and specificity, and is the diagnostic method of choice. Findings during endoscopy include white or yellow colored plaques, which, on subsequent histologic examination, demonstrate epithelial, fungal, bacterial, and inflammatory cells. Ulcerations are rarely seen but may occur in neutropenic patients. Brushings usually provide a higher diagnostic value; preparation of biopsies for histologic examination may lead to loss of organisms thereby affecting the results.

Therapy

General supportive therapy with intravenous hydration and nutritional support should be considered for patients who cannot eat or drink because of severe symptoms. In AIDS patients, use of highly active anti-retroviral therapy to increase the CD4 count results in clinical improvement.

Oral therapy, primarily with the azole antifungals, and intravenous therapy, mainly with amphotericin B, are used in the treatment of candida esophagitis. Oral therapy is used for immunocompetent patients, and immunocompromised patients without neutropenia who are able to tolerate oral feeding. Intravenous therapy is reserved for patients who cannot take medications by mouth, and neutropenic patients in whom the risk of disseminated candidiasis is high.

Specifically, immunocompetent patients, mildly immunocompromised patients, and AIDS patients should all be treated with fluconazole at 100 mg given orally every day for 2 weeks, with a 200 mg loading dose given on day one. Studies have demonstrated this regimen to be superior to treatment with ketoconazole, and equivalent to itraconazole solution given at 200 mg p.o. daily. The advantages of fluconazole are non-pH dependent or meal-dependent absorption, and its availability in intravenous or oral form. The major side effects of azole therapy are dose-dependent nausea and liver toxicity, and inhibition of cyclosporin metabolism, an important concern when used in transplant patients.

Amphotericin B, at a dose of 0.5 mg per kg per day given intravenously, should be used in neutropenic patients who are at higher risk for disseminated disease, patients who cannot tolerate oral medications, and patients with disease refractory to azole therapy. Amphotericin B is the most effective treatment; it offers a 95% cure rate with a 7-day course of therapy in AIDS patients, compared to an 80% cure rate with fluconazole. Severe side effects, especially renal toxicity, limit its routine use.

Flucytosine, another antifungal medication, can be used in conjunction with either amphotericin B or itraconazole, but large trials examining its efficacy are lacking. One small trial compared standard amphotericin B with amphotericin B fat emulsion in the treatment of candidal esophagitis in AIDS patients. The results showed similar clinical and microbiological efficacy; however, use of amphotericin B fat emulsion preparation was associated with a more favorable side-effect profile.

Antifungal resistance

If resistance to azole antifungals is suspected, increasing the dose of the azole may be tried. If this fails, changing to another azole may be attempted. If both tactics do not result in clinical improvement, use of intravenous amphotericin can achieve a cure in 90% of patients. For example, an AIDS patient with candida esophagitis treated initially with fluconazole, 100 mg p.o. daily fails to respond. The dose of fluconazole may be increased to 200 mg p.o. daily. If the patient fails to respond to the increased dose, itraconazole solution, 200 mg p.o. daily, may be used (perhaps in conjunction with flucytosine at a dose of 50 to 150 mg per kg daily, divided into four doses). If the patient fails to respond again, intravenous amphotericin may be used. It is important to ensure that an alternate or co-existing diagnosis is not overlooked.

Resistance to azole antifungals is related to prior exposure to azoles, and a CD4 count less than 50 per mm³. Resistance to amphotericin B is rare. Susceptibility testing may be helpful to isolate resistant strains and to determine susceptibility profile.

Prophylaxis

Although routine prophylaxis is unnecessary, it may be considered for patients with advanced AIDS and severe, recurrent esophagitis. Fluconazole 50 mg taken orally daily is effective for prophylaxis.

Herpes simplex virus esophagitis

Epidemiology

Herpes simplex virus type 1 is the second most common cause of infectious esophagitis. In the immunocompetent population HSV esophagitis is rare and may represent acute HSV infection or reactivation disease. The mean age of onset is 29 years old, and in patients less than 40 years of age, 77% are male and 23% are female. In patients older than 40 years of age there is no sex predominance.

In patients with HIV, HSV esophagitis is also relatively infrequent; cases of CMV esophagitis outnumber HSV esophagitis by two to one. HSV esophagitis may co-exist with candida esophagitis in AIDS patients. However, in transplant patients receiving immunosuppressive medications, the HSV and CMV esophagitis occur with equal frequency. Herpes simplex virus esophagitis is summarized in Box 2.3.

Clinical manifestations

The most common symptoms associated with HSV esophagitis are acute odynophagia, dysphagia, and substernal chest pain. Sometimes, a prodrome of systemic symptoms, such as fever and sore throat, may precede the esophageal symptoms. Other less common symptoms may include nausea, vomiting, epigastric pain, and heartburn.

Box 2.3 Herpes simplex virus (HSV) esophagitis

Epidemiology
Second most common cause of infectious esophagitis.
AIDS patients: CMV esophagitis > HSV esophagitis.
Transplant patients: HSV esophagitis = CMV esophagitis.

Symptoms and signs
Sudden onset of odynophagia.
May also have dysphagia, substernal chest pain, and oral ulcers.
Prodrome of fever and sore throat may occur.

Diagnosis
Upper endoscopy with biopsy and brushings is the optimal test:
   grossly, may see ulcers, most often affects the distal esophagus
   take biopsies from the edge of the ulcer
   send for histology, viral culture, immunohistochemistry.

Therapy
Immunocompetent host:
   symptomatic treatment with topical anesthetics and oral analgesics
   consider acyclovir 400 mg p.o. five times per day.
Immunocompromised host:
   acyclovir 400 mg p.o. 5 times per day for mild cases in patients tolerating oral medicines.
   acyclovir 5 mg/kg every 8 hours for 7–10 days for severe cases, and for patients not tolerating oral medications.
Acyclovir-resistant cases:
   foscarnet 40 mg/kg i.v. every 8 hours.

The physical examination may sometimes reveal oral ulcers, or evidence of complications, including bleeding, or tracheo-esophageal fistulas.

Diagnosis

Barium esophagram may show small shallow ulcers in up to 87% of patients. In 97% of cases, multiple ulcers are present involving large segments of the esophagus. Cobblestoning and a shaggy mucosal appearance are other possible findings. Compared to immunocompromised patients, immunocompetent patients typically have less extensive ulcerations and esophageal involvement.

Upper endoscopy with biopsy and brushings is the diagnostic test of choice. The biopsy and brushings should be performed at the ulcer edge, where the cytopathic effects occur. At the time of endoscopy, greater than 80% of patients will have ulcerations and friable mucosa. Deep ulcers are rare, and should suggest alternate diagnoses. About 40% will have whitish exudates. The distal esophagus is affected in about two-thirds of cases. The infection is generally limited to the squamous mucosa, and progresses from vesicle formation to ulceration, and eventually to coalescing ulcers. Tissue should be sent for immunohistochemical staining, viral culture, and histology. Histology will typically show multinucleated giant cells, and ground glass nuclei with eosinophilic inclusions (Cowdry type A inclusion bodies). Histology and viral culture will yield a diagnosis of HSV esophagitis in 97% of cases.

Therapy

Therapy for HSV esophagitis in the immunocompetent host is controversial. Given that most cases will resolve spontaneously in approximately 2 weeks, some authorities have advocated symptomatic treatment with topical analgesics such as viscous lidocaine or oral analgesics. However, others argue that antiviral therapy may decrease the duration of symptoms, and with the safety profile of acyclovir, all patients, including immunocompetent patients, should be treated. The dose of acyclovir is 400 mg taken orally five times per day for 14 days. In immunocompetent patients with severe symptoms and no oral intake, acyclovir, 5 mg per kg of body weight given intravenously every 8 hours, may be used.

No prospective, randomized, controlled trials have been performed to compare the benefits and risks of symptomatic treatment and antiviral therapy.

In immunosuppressed patients, treatment with acyclovir is indicated. In patients with limited immunosuppression, with mild symptoms, oral acyclovir (at a dose of 400 mg orally five times a day for 14 days) may be used. However, patients with significant immunosuppression or severe symptoms, or who cannot take oral medications, should be treated with intravenous acyclovir, 5 mg per kg of body weight every 8 hours for 7 to 10 days. Foscarnet (40 mg per kg given intravenously every 8 hours) may be used for acyclovir-resistant cases of HSV esophagitis.

Prophylaxis

AIDS patients with relapsing disease may benefit from acyclovir prophylaxis given as 400 mg orally twice a day. The same regimen may benefit HSV-positive post-transplantation patients with recurring disease.

Cytomegalovirus esophagitis

Epidemiology

Cytomegalovirus esophagitis, and CMV disease in general, primarily occurs in immunocompromised patients. With greater than 50% of the population in developed countries, and 90% of homosexual men seropositive for CMV, the disease is almost always due to reactivation during immunosuppression. In contrast, the immunocompetent patient may develop CMV esophagitis during primary CMV infection or during disease reactivation.

In immunosuppressed post-transplant patients not receiving antiviral prophylaxis, CMV is the most common opportunistic pathogen, and a major cause of morbidity and mortality. The risk of development of CMV disease in general is highest in lung and heart-lung transplant patients, with a prevalence of up to 75%. The risk of CMV disease is highest in CMV seronegative patients who receive an organ from a CMV seropositive donor. Use of antilymphocyte antibodies to treat organ rejection is also linked to higher risk of CMV disease. The risk of CMV disease is highest 1 to 4 months after transplantation. In the post-transplant patient, CMV and HSV esophagitis occur with equal frequency.

However, in AIDS patients, CMV is the most common cause of esophageal ulcers, and occurs with much greater frequency than HSV esophagitis. Cytomegalovirus esophagitis usually occurs when the CD4 count falls below 50 per mm^3. Cytomegalovirus esophagitis is summarized in Box 2.4.

Clinical manifestations

Patients with CMV esophagitis present with severe odynophagia and may have evidence of CMV infection in other organs. In AIDS patients, CMV retinitis often co-exists; AIDS patients with gastrointestinal CMV involvement should be examined by an ophthalmologist for retinal involvement. Complications of CMV esophagitis include hemorrhage, stricture, and fistula formation.

Diagnosis

Barium esophagram of patients with CMV esophagitis typically reveals the presence of large, single ulcers; occasionally, multiple ulcers may be seen. Deeper ulcerations are found in AIDS patients, and more superficial ulcerations are seen in non–AIDS patients. Ulcers in AIDS patients may be more than 2 cm in size.

Upper endoscopy with brushings and biopsy is the diagnostic test of choice. On visual inspection, multiple shallow ulcers, or single deeper ulcers may be seen. Unlike diagnosis of HSV esophagitis, biopsies for diagnosis of CMV esophagitis are best taken from

---

Box 2.4 Cytomegalovirus (CMV) esophagitis

Epidemiology
Primarily occurs in immunocompromised hosts.
Most of the population is CMV seropositive.
It is the most common opportunistic pathogen in post-transplant patients who are not receiving prophylaxis.
Risk for CMV esophagitis in AIDS patients increases when CD4 counts are less than 50/m^3.

Symptoms and signs
Severe odynophagia.
There may be CMV involvement of other organs.
AIDS patients may have concurrent CMV retinitis.

Diagnosis
Upper endoscopy with biopsy and brushings is the optimal test:
    grossly, may see ulcers (ulcers are deeper in AIDS patients)
    take at least ten biopsies from the base of the ulcer
    send for immunohistochemistry and viral culture examination for cytopathic effect.

Therapy
Active disease:
    ganciclovir 5 mg/kg i.v. every 12 hours for 21 days
    post-transplant patients may benefit from maintenance therapy
    ganciclovir 5 mg per kg i.v. daily for 3 to 6 weeks, or
    ganciclovir 1000 mg p.o. t.i.d. for 3 to 6 weeks.
Prophylaxis in transplant patients:
    ganciclovir 1000 mg p.o. t.i.d. for 3 to 6 months
    intravenous ganciclovir in various protocols.

---

the ulcer base. For the highest diagnostic yield, at least ten biopsies should be taken and sent for immunohistochemistry, viral culture, and examination for cytopathic effect. The cytopathic effect induced by CMV is seen in the endothelium and granulation tissue, in contrast to the squamous mucosal involvement in HSV esophagitis. Mucosal damage is thought to be secondary to ischemia resulting from endothelial damage and disruption of the vascular supply. Histologic examination may show large, eosinophilic inclusions in the nucleus and cytoplasm.

Therapy

First-line therapy for CMV esophagitis is the intravenous administration of ganciclovir. AIDS patient should receive 5 mg per kg given twice a day for 21 days; this regimen has a 77% response rate. Institution of highly active anti-retroviral therapy to increase the CD4 count is an important part of treatment.

Although no formal recommendations exist, therapy of CMV esophagitis in post-transplant recipients involves prevention of CMV disease in the immediate post-transplant period, and treatment of active CMV disease. Both oral and intravenous long-term ganciclovir therapy have been used for the prevention of CMV disease in the post-transplant period. Intravenous therapy with ganciclovir 2.5 mg per kg given daily to renal-transplant patients receiving anti-lymphocyte antibody treatment for rejection lowered the incidence of CMV disease in these patients. Intravenous ganciclovir administered to liver-transplant recipients at a dose of 6 mg per kg given daily for 1 month, followed by 6 mg per kg given five times a week for another 70 days lowered CMV infection rates when compared to acyclovir. Oral ganciclovir at 1000 mg given three times daily has been used in high-risk liver- or kidney-transplant patients (CMV seropositive donor, CMV seronegative recipient, use of anti-lymphocyte antibodies for rejection) for 3 to 6 months. Patients receiving ganciclovir have been shown to exhibit statistically significant lower rates of CMV disease when compared to patients receiving acyclovir (studies done with renal-transplant patients), or placebo

(studies done with liver-transplant patients). Specific prophylactic regimens should be tailored to the individual patient, and should be consistent with institutional recommendations.

Treatment of active CMV esophagitis in the post-transplant patient is similar to treatment for all active CMV esophagitis, and is accomplished with intravenous ganciclovir, 5 mg per kg every 12 hours for 3 weeks. However, because the relapse rate approaches 40%, some experts have advocated the use of 3 to 6 weeks of maintenance therapy (with intravenous ganciclovir, 5 mg per kg given daily, or oral ganciclovir, 1000 mg given three times a day) to prevent recurrence, particularly in the CMV seropositive donor, CMV seronegative recipient population. Patients who do not respond to the initial treatment with ganciclovir may benefit from immunosuppression reduction, use of CMV immune globulin, or sensitivity testing for ganciclovir resistance.

In patients with ganciclovir-resistant CMV esophagitis foscarnet, 90 to 120 mg per kg, should be given intravenously every day.

Esophagitis in the AIDS patient

Epidemiology

Forty per cent of patients with AIDS are affected by esophagitis in the course of their illness; candida esophagitis accounts for greater than 50% of esophagitis in this population. The remainder of cases are composed of HSV, CMV, Kaposi's sarcoma, and idiopathic esophageal ulcers. Symptoms attributable to esophagitis are the second most common gastrointestinal symptom after diarrhea.

Approach to diagnosis and therapy

The approach to esophagitis in AIDS patients is summarized in Figure 2.1. AIDS patients with esophagitis typically present with odynophagia,

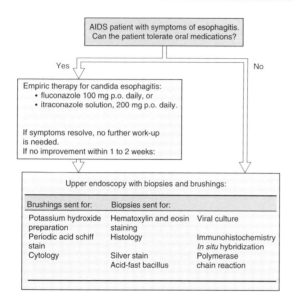

Figure 2.1 Approach to esophagitis in the AIDS patient.

dysphagia, and substernal chest pain. Because candida esophagitis accounts for greater than half of all cases, initial empiric treatment with fluconazole 100 mg p.o. daily may be tried. If the patient cannot take oral medications, or if there is no clinical response in one or two weeks, further diagnostic workup should be performed.

Upper endoscopy with biopsies and brushings should be done. White plaques or exudates suggest candida esophagitis (which, with no clinical response, may be resistant to fluconazole). Ulcerations and erosions suggest viral esophagitis. Brushings and biopsies should be sent for KOH prep, PAS staining, and cytology if fungal esophagitis is suggested; other tests that should be performed in the appropriate clinical settings are H and E staining, AFB testing, silver staining, histology, immuno-histochemistry, PCR and in-situ hybridization, and viral cultures.

Keeping a broad differential diagnosis is important. Aside from infectious etiologies, esophageal symptoms in AIDS patients may also be caused by medications and malignancies (such as lymphoma).

Other causes of infectious esophagitis

Fungal

Esophagitis caused by non-candida fungi is a rare occurrence. Esophageal involvement by histoplasmosis, aspergillosis, blastomycosis, and mucormycosis have been reported.

Histoplasma capsulatum-induced esophageal disease usually occurs as a complication of pulmonary histoplasmosis with mediastinal involvement and subsequent extension to the esophagus. However, primary esophageal histoplasmosis has been reported in patients with HIV, immunocompromised status (most commonly due to glucocorticoid use), diabetes mellitus, and GERD. Diagnosis of secondary histoplasmosis should be through computed tomography (CT) of the chest, demonstrating pulmonary or mediastinal involvement; in these patients, endoscopy is often negative due to lack of squamous mucosal involvement. Primary esophageal histoplasmosis may be diagnosed via endoscopy.

Esophagitis caused by *Aspergillus* species may be diagnosed with endoscopy. Cytology performed on esophageal brushings may demonstrate the septate hyphae of *Aspergillus* species, and fungal culture may confirm the diagnosis.

Histoplasmosis and blastomycosis may be treated with ketoconazole, itraconazole, or amphotericin B. Aspergillus should be treated with high-dose amphotericin B.

Mycobacterial

Mycobacterial esophageal infection is rare in both immunocompetent and immunocompromised patients, and occurs frequently with *Mycobacterium tuberculosis* (TB) than with *Mycobacterium avium* complex (MAC). The esophagus is most commonly involved secondarily through fistulization with mediastinal lymph nodes or via direct extension from a pharyngeal or upper airway source.

Patients may experience symptoms of dysphagia, or may have respiratory difficulties if fistulas to the pulmonary tract are present. Hemoptysis or hematemesis may also occur. Upper endoscopy with brushings and biopsies will usually reveal the diagnosis.

Treatment with anti-TB regimens, or with clarithromycin and ethambutol for MAC will usually result in clinical improvement.

Bacterial

Bacterial esophagitis is rare and tends to affect patients who have hematologic malignancies accompanied by neutropenia, who are status post-bone marrow transplantation, and who are in diabetic ketoacidosis.

The organisms most commonly implicated in bacterial esophagitis are oral flora, including *Streptococcus viridans* and *Staphylococcus* spp. Organisms causing disease in AIDS patients include *Bartonella* spp., *Actinomyces* spp., and *Nocardia* spp. Bacteria cause local infection by invading mucosa that has been compromised by chemotherapy or radiation therapy. Neutropenic patients are at risk for systemic dissemination.

Endoscopic findings include ulcers, erythema, pseudomembranes, and hemorrhage. Sulfur granules may be associated with actinomyces infection. Diagnosis is established through Gram's stain and culture. Blood cultures may also be helpful.

Initial empiric antibiotic therapy should cover oropharyngeal flora, and then tailored to the specific organism once culture and sensitivity results are available.

Pill-induced esophagitis

Background

Epidemiology

With the increasing prescription of medications in medical practice, the recognition of pill-induced esophagitis is becoming increasingly important. In fact, over 1000 cases of pill-induced esophagitis have been reported in the medical literature over the last 30 years, and the actual number of cases may be higher because of underreporting.

Epidemiologically, females are affected more often than males, in a ratio of 2:1, perhaps reflecting the increased usage of potentially harmful medications such as alendronate, antibiotics, and NSAIDs by women. Although the classic case involves a patient who spontaneously presents with a sudden onset of odynophagia and pain, some risk factors for pill-induced esophagitis have been identified. The most common locations for development of esophagitis are at the level of the aortic arch (the junction of the proximal third with the middle third of the esophagus), the gastroesophageal junction, and the level of the left atrium. Pill-induced esophagitis is summarized in Box 2.5.

Risk factors

Any behavior that prolongs esophageal transit time may increase the risk of injury. Assuming a supine position immediately, or shortly after, pill ingestion eliminates the positional effect of gravity as a factor in esophageal clearance. Ingesting pills before bedtime increases esophageal transit time because salivation and swallowing frequency are decreased during sleep. Inadequate liquid intake after pill ingestion promotes retention of the pill in the esophagus. Patients older than 70 years of age have decreased amplitude of peristaltic

Box 2.5 Pill-induced esophagitis

Epidemiology
Females are affected more often than males.
Most common locations are the level of the
  aortic arch and level of the left atrium.
Most commonly implicated medications:
  antibiotics – doxycycline, tetracycline
  NSAIDs – aspirin, naproxen sodium,
    ibuprofen, indometacin
  cardiac medications – potassium chloride,
    quinidine
  alendronate

Risk factors
Inadequate liquid intake or lying supine after
  pill ingestion.
Age over 70 years.
History of thoracic surgery or cardiac disease.

Symptoms and signs
Severe odynophagia and retrosternal pain.
Dysphagia should suggest an alternate diagnosis.

Diagnosis
No testing necessary in classic cases without
  symptoms or signs of complications.
Work up atypical or severe cases with an upper
  gastrointestinal series or upper endoscopy
  (the most sensitive test).

Prevention
Take medications with more than 150 ml
  water and remain upright for 10 minutes.
Patients using alendronate should take
  medication with 250 ml water and remain
  upright for 30 minutes.

Treatment
Most will heal in a few weeks.
No proven benefit from H_2 blockers, proton
  pump inhibitors, or sucralfate.
Supportive care with hydration and
  nutrition as needed.
Consider dilation in patients with strictures.

example, studies have shown that larger pills have a longer transit time in the esophagus than smaller pills. Gelatinous pills also tend to stick to the esophageal mucosa more often than those with other types of coating. Some studies suggest that sustained-release preparations have an increased risk of causing esophagitis when compared with normal-release preparations of the same medications.

Certain anatomical factors may predispose to pill-induced esophagitis. Patients who have had a thoracotomy are at increased risk. Normally, the esophagus has mobility within the thorax, moving to allow passage of food and other swallowed substances. After thoracotomy, adhesions may develop in the mediastinum, causing the esophagus' position in the chest to be relatively fixed, compounding the effects of other potential risk factors such as an increased left atrial size or aortic arch entrapment.

Patients with a history of cardiac disease are also at higher risk for development of pill-induced esophagitis. These patients may use more medications that are known to cause esophagitis, such as aspirin, potassium chloride, and quinidine. They may also have a larger left atrium than the general population, because of valvular heart disease or congestive heart failure. Since the left atrium lies anterior to the esophagus in the mediastinum, an enlarged left atrial size may compress the esophagus posteriorly. The compression interferes with the passage of swallowed items such as medications.

Surprisingly, pre-existing esophageal motility disorders have not been shown to be a risk factor for pill-induced esophagitis. Perhaps these patients are more careful and drink more liquids after swallowing their medications.

contractions, which may lead to increased esophageal transit times and inefficient clearance of medications.

Certain characteristics of the medication itself may increase the risk of esophagitis. For

Pathogenesis

Although medications may cause esophageal injury through systemic effects such as decreasing the resting pressure of the lower esophageal sphincter, we will discuss only esophagitis caused by direct injury to the esophagus by the medication.

During pill ingestion, the medication comes into contact with the esophageal mucosa for a surprisingly long period of time.

The patient's position during and following pill ingestion is a major determinant of esophageal transit time. In one study normal subjects were asked to swallow barium sulfate tablets with 15 ml of water, and then lie down. The barium sulfate tablets were shown to be retained in the esophagus for up to 5 minutes. Another study demonstrated that gelatin capsules ingested while supine, with or without water, remained in the esophagus for longer than 10 minutes in over half the subjects, whereas the same pills ingested while upright with 15 ml of water were rapidly cleared.

The quantity of water taken with the medication also contributes to esophageal clearance. One study demonstrated that gelatin capsules swallowed with 15 ml of water became trapped at the level of the aortic arch in 39% of subjects, and at the gastroesophageal junction in 22% of subjects. When the same capsules were swallowed with 120 ml of water, only one subject experienced entrapment of the capsule at the aortic arch, and only two subjects had lodging of the capsule at the gastroesophageal junction.

These studies demonstrate that pill ingestion while supine or with insufficient water bolus increases esophageal transit time, and predisposes the patient to pill-induced esophagitis. Regardless of the cause, prolonged contact of the pill with the esophageal mucosa may cause injury by various proposed mechanisms.

Some medications, such as tetracyclines, ascorbic acid, and ferrous sulfate, produce an acidic solution when mixed with water or saliva. Other medications, including phenytoin sodium, result in an alkaline solution under similar conditions. Contact with the esophageal mucosa may result in an acidic or alkaline burn.

Other medications such as potassium chloride do not cause a pH change, but result in a local hyperosmolar state, which may cause tissue injury via cellular dessication.

Medications such as doxycycline and non-steroidal anti-inflammatory drugs (NSAIDs) are taken up by esophageal mucosa, and may cause toxic damage to the mucosa directly.

Diagnosis

History and physical examination

The classic presentation of pill-induced esophagitis is a patient (particularly a young patient taking tetracycline for treatment of acne) without a previous history of esophageal disorders who presents with a sudden onset of retrosternal pain and odynophagia. The patient may say that a pill "got stuck" during swallowing in the recent past. The degree of pain may vary, and may be so severe as to prevent swallowing, leading to weight loss and dehydration. If the patient took the pill at night or before assuming a supine position, he or she may report that the pain awakened them from sleep. Older patients may confuse the pain from esophagitis with cardiac angina; in patients with significant risk factors, a cardiac disorder should be ruled out. The pain typically worsens over a period of 3 to 4 days, then gradually improves.

Obvious risk factors should be sought out in the history. The patient should be asked if he or she recently took a pill before bedtime or before assuming a supine position. The amount of liquid intake after medication ingestion should be determined. A history of thoracic surgery or heart disease, and a list of the patient's medications should be obtained. Certain medications have a greater incidence of specific complications. For example, NSAID-induced esophagitis may be complicated by hemorrhage, while potassium chloride esophagitis may be complicated by strictures.

Although it may occur with potassium chloride, ferrous sulfate, or quinidine, dysphagia is uncommon, and should suggest a stricture complicating esophagitis or an alternate diagnosis, such as malignancy.

Studies

The diagnosis should be suggested by a history of implicated medication use, and the presence of risk factors. In classic cases, no further testing may be necessary. However, if the presentation is atypical (raising the suspicion of possible alternate diagnoses) or suggests a complication or an unusual degree of severity, additional diagnostic studies with an upper endoscopy or an upper gastrointestinal series may be warranted.

Upper endoscopy is the most sensitive procedure; virtually 100% of patients will have abnormal findings. In patients with severe, persistent, or progressive symptoms, upper endoscopy is indicated to determine the degree of severity and presence of complications, and to rule out alternate diagnoses. When dysphagia is the predominant symptom, an upper endoscopy may help to assess the presence of strictures or malignancy. Patients with signs or symptoms of upper gastrointestinal hemorrhage should have an upper endoscopy to look for perforation or major vessel involvement by erosion. In immunocompromised patients, an upper endoscopy may exclude other possible diagnoses such as infectious esophagitis. Performing biopsies and brushings of the esophagus at the time of upper endoscopy may reveal alternative diagnoses such as GERD, neoplastic disorders, and infectious diseases.

Useful findings at the time of endoscopy include location, appearance, and presence or absence of complications. The most common areas for pill esophagitis to occur are at the level of the aortic arch, at the level of the left atrium in patients with left atrial enlargement, and at the gastroesophageal junction. Typically, a discrete ulcer of variable size (from 1 or 2 mm to a few cm in size) may be seen. The ulcer may be surrounded by normal mucosa. Sometimes, multiple ulcers may be present, and the ulcer(s) may contain pill remnants. With regard to complications, hemorrhage or strictures may also be visualized by upper endoscopy, and therapy for these complications may be initiated at that time.

Because some medications such as NSAIDs, quinidine, and ferrous sulfate may cause nodular inflammation and exudate, a biopsy with brushings may be used to exclude malignancy or infection. Biopsies, however, are not always necessary, and in routine cases usually only show inflammatory changes. The damage is usually limited to mucosa, although deeper involvement may occur.

An upper gastrointestinal series is not as sensitive as upper endoscopy for the assessment of pill-induced esophagitis, but can be utilized to look for extrinsic compression, neoplasia, and the presence of foreign bodies. Only double contrast technique should be used to visualize the ulcer.

A possible approach to the patient begins with the history and physical examination. If the patient gives a typical history, the pain is not severe, and no complications are suggested, therapy may be initiated without further testing. However, if alternate diagnoses are possible, if the pain is severe, or if complications may exist, an upper gastrointestinal series may be performed. In cases where the patient complains of dysphagia or bleeding, patient fails conservative management, or is immunocompromised, an upper endoscopy should be performed.

Therapy

Prevention

The most effective approach to pill-induced esophagitis is prevention through patient education and avoidance of potentially caustic medications in patients at risk for esophagitis. Pills should be taken with at least 150 ml of water (250 ml if using alendronate), and the patient should remain upright for at least 10 minutes after medication ingestion (30 minutes if using alendronate). For patients who remain supine, such as elderly nursing-home patients, medications may be given in liquid form or suspension form.

Treatment

Most cases of pill-induced esophagitis will heal spontaneously in a few weeks. Adjunctive therapy with antacids, H_2 blockers, proton pump inhibitors, and sucralfate are used, but do not have a proven benefit. These medications may have a role in cases of distal esophageal injury and NSAID-induced esophagitis to prevent exacerbation by acid reflux.

Patients who have severe odynophagia accompanied by weight loss and dehydration should be treated with intravenous hydration, and if their condition does not improve within a few days, with parenteral nutrition.

Serious, life-threatening hemorrhage is rare but may occur, particularly with NSAID-induced esophagitis, and should be treated in an intensive care setting. Volume expansion should be accomplished with crystalloid and appropriate blood products. Upper endoscopy should be performed to assess the location of hemorrhage, and provide treatment if possible. Surgical consultation should be obtained in such circumstances.

Esophageal strictures should be suspected in patients who complain of dysphagia. Strictures may be a late sequelae of esophagitis, or may be found at the time of initial presentation. Endoscopic dilation should be attempted for chronic strictures, and if unsuccessful, surgical bypass may be considered but is rarely needed.

Specific causes of pill-induced esophagitis

Antibiotics

A recent literature review identified antibiotics as causing roughly 50% of cases of pill-induced esophagitis. Tetracycline, doxycycline, and other related compounds accounted for approximately 80% of antibiotic associated cases. Patients with esophagitis caused by antibiotic use usually present with severe, acute pain from mucosal ulceration. They are usually young, with no other predisposing risk factors or esophageal disorders. Strictures rarely develop in these cases, since the severe pain brings the patient to medical attention promptly, and because the pill remnants are rapidly cleared from the esophagus.

Anti-inflammatory agents

Non-steroidal anti-inflammatory drugs comprise slightly less than 10% of cases of pill-induced esophagitis, but account for 50% of cases of pill-induced esophageal hemorrhage. In fact, one out of four cases of NSAID-induced esophagitis is complicated by esophageal hemorrhage. Aspirin, naproxen sodium, ibuprofen, and indomethacin are common culprits, perhaps reflecting their widespread use; in contrast, selective COX 2 inhibitors may possess a lower risk of esophagitis. Patients may present with symptoms of heartburn, regurgitation, and dysphagia; some patients have also developed ulcers or bleeding without warning. Others may present with stricture formation. Unlike patients with antibiotic-associated esophagitis, patients with NSAID-induced esophageal injury often have co-existent disorders, including GERD, hiatal hernia, esophageal rings, or esophageal dysmotility. Some have postulated an association between patients with reflux disease and the development of esophageal strictures with NSAID use.

Non-steroidal anti-inflammatory drugs damage the esophageal mucosa through a few different mechanisms, they are weak organic acids and may cause a pH-mediated caustic injury. Additionally, they may also decrease esophageal resistance to gastric acid by disrupting the mucosal barrier. This effect is greater when aspirin is combined with alcohol. Also, in patients with GERD, NSAIDs are absorbed into the esophageal mucosa, directly causing inflammation.

Prevention of NSAID-induced esophagitis follows the same principles as those outlined above. Pills should be taken with one large glass of water, preferably 1 hour before bedtime in the upright position. Liquid forms of the medications should be used (if possible) in bedridden patients, and patients with pre-existing esophageal motility disorders.

Cardiac medications

Potassium chloride-induced esophagitis has a different clinical course to that induced by the agents mentioned above. Approximately 80% of cases occurred in patients with extrinsic compression of the esophagus or esophageal motor dysfunction. Almost two-thirds of cases occurred in patients with a prior history of cardiac surgery, which predisposes to esophageal entrapment between the aorta and the vertebrae because of adhesion formation. Sustained-release formulations of potassium chloride cause esophagitis more often than immediate-release formulations. Lesions caused by potassium chloride usually cause little pain. Therefore, patients continue to take potassium chloride tablets because of a lack of early warning symptoms. The esophageal injury progresses, resulting in stricture formation and progressive dysphagia. Unlike NSAID-induced esophagitis, hemorrhage rarely occurs.

Quinidine-induced esophagitis is associated with the formation of a profuse, irregular exudate that adheres to the esophageal mucosa. Its appearance as a filling defect on upper gastrointestinal series may suggest malignancy, prompting an upper endoscopy with biopsy. Only two patients with quinidine-induced esophagitis had a predisposing risk factor. Quinidine was also associated with stricture formation in over 50% of cases.

Alendronate

Initial studies of alendronate demonstrated that 199 of 475 000 patients developed esophagitis, 51 of whom had severe effects, and 32 of whom required hospitalization. Esophagitis was more common in patients with pre-existing esophageal disorders. Upper endoscopy revealed erosions, ulcerations, and exudate formation, sometimes involving more than 10 cm of mucosa; bleeding, however, was rare. Further analysis of this study showed that more than half of the patients did not take alendronate with sufficient water, or did not remain upright for 30 minutes after ingestion.

A later study that followed 994 patients for 3 years of therapy with alendronate found no increased risk of esophagitis over placebo when the medication was taken in the upright position with sufficient water intake. The results were attributed to improved patient education and instruction, and frequent follow-up visits.

Overall recommendations are that patients should take alendronate with 150 ml of water, and remain upright for 30 minutes. Alendronate should be used with caution in patients with pre-existing esophageal disorders, and should be discontinued in patients who develop esophagitis.

Corrosive esophagitis

Background

Most instances of corrosive esophagitis occur in children. Children ingest household chemicals accidentally, and may subsequently expectorate much of the substance, limiting the amount of damage to the esophagus. However, in the remainder of cases, adolescents and adults attempting suicide swallow larger amounts of caustic materials without expectoration, leading to greater trauma.

The insult typically happens at the level of the aortic arch, the narrowest region of the esophagus. The degree of injury is related to the inherent properties of the substance (most important of which is pH), the speed at which it is cleared from the esophagus, the concentration and state (solid or liquid) of the substance, and the amount consumed. Liquid agents may cause widespread damage as it coats the esophageal mucosa, while solids tend to stick to the mucosa, causing localized injury. The two major categories of caustic substances are alkalis, such as lye and dishwashing detergents, and acids in cleaning solutions. Corrosive esophagitis is summarized in Box 2.6.

Causes

Alkali

Alkalis that may harm the esophagus include sodium or potassium hydroxide chemicals (collectively known as "lye"), detergents, such as dishwashing fluid, and button batteries. Button batteries can cause burns in 4 hours, and perforation within 6 hours, as well as pressure necrosis and electrical injury. The requisite pH for injury is thought to be 12.5.

Alkaline damage to the esophagus results in liquifactive necrosis, which occurs in seconds. Liquifactive necrosis will then progress to mucosal ulceration and sloughing within a few days, leading to thinning of the esophageal wall within 2 weeks, and ultimately to fibrosis and re-epithelialization in a couple of months. Severe cases may progress rapidly or indolently to esophageal perforation, mediastinitis, and death.

Box 2.6 Corrosive esophagitis

Epidemiology
Most often occurs in children.
In children it is usually accidental ingestion.
In adults it is often a suicide attempt.
Damage occurs at the level of the aortic arch.
Alkalis cause more damage than acids.

Symptoms and signs
Symptoms of pain, odynophagia, dysphagia, hypersalivation, severity of symptoms does not not correlate to extent of damage.
Back pain, retrosternal pain, peritoneal signs, or crepitus suggest esophageal perforation.
Dyspnea, stridor, or hoarseness suggest upper airway involvement.

Diagnosis
Plain films may help to rule out perforation.
Upper endoscopy helps to assess damage and determine prognosis.

Therapy
Initiate basic assessment and management of airway, breathing, and circulation.
Patient should be made nothing by mouth.
No role for lavage, induced vomiting, or chemical neutralization of caustic substance.
Possible role for placement of nasogastric tube to maintain esophageal patency for future stricture dilation therapy.
Treat long-term complications such as strictures, loss of peristalsis, and increased incidence of gastroesophageal reflux disease.

Acids

Acidic substances induce less esophageal damage than alkaline substances. Acids cause more pain on ingestion, which may limit the amount ingested. In addition, salivary bicarbonate may neutralize a portion of the acid ingested. Because most acidic substances are less viscous in their liquid form than alkali, they are cleared faster by the esophagus, limiting the duration of mucosal contact.

Acid-induced damage takes longer to occur, and results in coagulation necrosis. In contrast to liquifactive necrosis caused by alkali which may spread rapidly to involve all layers of the esophageal wall, coagulation necrosis creates an eschar over the affected region, effectively limiting injury to submucosal tissues.

Diagnosis

History and physical examination

Although symptoms of pain, dysphagia, odynophagia, hypersalivation, and drooling may indicate significant injury, a lack of overt symptoms, particularly in children, does not rule out severe injury. Back or retrosternal pain may signify esophageal perforation, while dyspnea, stridor, or hoarseness may suggest aspiration and upper airway involvement. Peritoneal signs or crepitus may occur in cases with esophageal perforation.

Studies

Abdominal or chest films may show evidence of pleural fluid, mediastinitis, or perforation.

All patients with symptoms of injury such as vomiting, dysphagia, odynophagia, abdominal pain, or oral pain, and patients with evidence of ingestion on examination, such as oral mucosal damage or drooling, should undergo an upper endoscopy. Upper endoscopy should be performed to assess the degree of damage and to guide further therapy; however, upper endoscopy is contraindicated in patients with evidence of perforation or hemodynamic instability. Upper endoscopy may show edema, hemorrhage, ulcerations, or mucosal sloughing, and may provide data to determine the extent of injury and guide treatment and prognosis. Examples of proposed endoscopic grading systems are given in Table 2.2.

Table 2.2 Examples of endoscopic grading systems in corrosive esophagitis

Based on depth of injury

1st degree	superficial injury with edema, hemorrhage: no scar formation.
2nd degree	ulcerations, exudates, and vesicle formation: scarring and stricture may occur.
3rd degree	necrosis, penetration of injury through esophageal wall: and/or perforation.

Based on gross endoscopic findings

Grade 0	normal
Grade 1	mucosal erythema and hyperemia: no significant morbidity or stricture risk.
Grade 2A	superficial ulcers, bleeding and exudates: no significant morbidity or stricture risk.
Grade 2B	deep focal or circumferential ulcers: 70%–100% stricture risk.
Grade 3A	focal necrosis: 70%–100% stricture risk.
Grade 3B	extensive necrosis: 65% early mortality, most will require esophageal resection and intestinal interposition.

Therapy

General management

Initial management includes assessment of airway, breathing, and circulation. Because of the potential for respiratory tract involvement, determination of the patient's airway patency and respiratory sufficiency is vital. If the epiglottis or larynx are involved, tracheostomy should be considered for airway management with appropriate surgical consultation. Symptoms and signs of hemodynamic instability should be sought and, if present, treatment with appropriate crystalloid resuscitation and blood-product infusion should be performed. If the patient is unstable, or the clinical assessment suggests severe injury, treatment in an intensive care setting may be appropriate.

In an asymptomatic patient who reports a reliable history of minimal ingestion without signs suggestive of deeper injury on examination, discharge and outpatient follow-up may be considered. For patients that do not meet these criteria, hospitalization (with potential intensive care admission for severe cases) is appropriate.

On admission, the patient should be made "nothing by mouth". Chest and abdominal films should be obtained; patients with signs or symptoms of perforation, such as peritonitis, free air on plain films, or mediastinitis should be managed with surgical consultation for urgent operative therapy. Unless contraindicated, upper endoscopy should be performed within 24 to 48 hours. As mentioned above, upper endoscopy helps to ascertain the extent of injury, guide therapy, and determine prognosis.

Specific therapy

There is no role for removal of the caustic agent by lavage, induced vomiting, or neutralization of the substance. These attempts may cause more mucosal injury. Induction of vomiting will increase damage by re-exposure of the mucosa to the caustic agent. Placement of a nasogastric or orogastric tube may cause emesis, or may perforate the weakened esophagus. However, some experts advocate the use of nasogastric tubes to maintain esophageal patency for future stricture dilation therapy. Use of neutralizing agents is not effective since damage has already been done. The chemical reaction of neutralization may release heat and result in thermal injury.

The role of steroids in management of caustic injury is controversial. There has been only one controlled trial which did not show benefit, although a retrospective literature review suggests a possible benefit in stricture prevention. However, other experts feel stricture formation is related only to the degree of injury. The role of broad spectrum antibiotics is also controversial.

Proton pump inhibitors may be useful to prevent superimposed GERD. For patients with severe injury, this may be required for several weeks and even months until adequate healing has occurred or the patient is amenable for surgery.

Long-term complications

Strictures occur in association with second and third degree injuries and circumferential injuries. They occur most commonly at the level of the aortic arch, and are usually long and rigid. Loss of distal esophageal peristalsis may lead to an increased risk of GERD and its complications, such as reflux esophagitis, strictures, Barrett's esophagus and potentially adenocarcinoma. Patients with distal esophageal dysmotility may require a proton pump inhibitor for aggressive anti-reflux treatment.

There is a one-thousand-fold increased risk of esophageal squamous cell carcinoma in patients with a history of lye ingestion when compared to the general population (baseline risk of esophageal squamous cell carcinoma is 2.6 cases per 100 000). The mean latency period is 41 years, with a range of 13 to 71 years. The latency period is shorter in patients exposed to lye later in life. The prognosis of esophageal squamous cell carcinoma in patients with lye exposure is slightly better than the general population. These patients present to medical attention sooner because scarring at the level of neoplasia causes dysphagia earlier in the disease course. In addition, esophageal scarring delays direct tumor extension and lymphatic spread.

Radiation esophagitis

Background

Despite attempts to shield the esophagus from radiation during therapy for malignancies such as lymphoma, lung cancer, or head and neck cancer, about one-half of patients will have some degree of esophagitis. Although formerly considered relatively radiation resistant, the esophagus may be damaged by radiation much like other stratified squamous epithelium. In addition, radiation also causes injury to the endothelium of vasculature within the esophagus. Radiation esophagitis is summarized in Box 2.7.

Pathogenesis

Squamous epithelium

Radiation suppresses the cell-proliferation in the basal layer of the epithelium by inhibiting germinal cell mitosis. Cells in the G1 phase of the cell cycle are particularly sensitive to radiation effects. Initially, cells may recover in a matter of days, but with repeated radiation exposure, cell damage may be permanent and lead to chronic damage. Following radiation exposure, the epithelium may slough off, leaving a denuded lamina propria. Additionally, loss of the protective epithelium may lead to decreased resistance to infection. Regeneration of the epithelium begins a few days after radiation treatment ceases, but may take a few months to reach maximal levels.

Endothelium

Inflammation, capillary dilation, and increased capillary permeability result in leukocyte

---

Box 2.7 Radiation esophagitis

Epidemiology
Occurs in 50% of patients receiving radiation
  therapy to the thorax or head and neck.
Damage occurs to both the squamous
  mucosa and endothelium.

Acute effects
Mucositis, dysphagia, odynophagia begin 2
  weeks after radiation exposure.
Hemorrhage and perforation are atypical; if
  present, pursue alternate diagnoses.

Chronic effects
Stricture formation due to fibrosis.
Fistulas and ulcerations which may lead to
  perforation.

Therapy
Acute effects:
    decrease daily radiation dose by 10%
    use topical anesthetic (viscous lidocaine) or
      systemic analgesic
    proton pump inhibitors or sucralfate may
      decrease pain exacerbated by
      gastroesophageal acid reflux.

Chronic effects:
limit total radiation exposure to less than
  60 Gy [conversion from 6000 rads to
  be confirmed]
use oblique or lateral fields to decrease
  esophageal radiation exposure
dilate or surgically bypass strictures
provide nutritional support.

migration, interstitial edema, and, grossly, erythema. Radiation may also induce thrombosis of blood vessels causing ischemia, tissue necrosis, and ulcer formation. Over time, continued thrombosis and resulting ischemia ultimately leads to epithelial atrophy and esophageal fibrosis.

Symptoms

Acute effects

Mucositis, dysphagia, and odynophagia begin to manifest by 2 weeks of radiation exposure. At 20 to 30 Gy (when administered at a rate of 1.8 to 2.0 Gy per day), patients may develop significant sharp chest pain radiating to the back. These symptoms typically last 24 to 48 hours, and may suggest a cardiac etiology. Symptoms begin to subside when therapy is temporarily stopped for 2 days, but it may take more than a week before they improve significantly. Hemorrhage and perforation are not typical of acute radiation esophagitis; if present, alternate diagnoses should be considered. Other physiological effects include an altered primary peristaltic wave and failure of LES relaxation.

Chronic effects

The potential for chronic esophageal damage depends on both the cumulative dose of radiation received and the length of esophagus exposed. The maximum tolerated dose is believed to be 60 Gy, delivered at a rate of 10 Gy per week; however, individual patient tolerances may vary. In addition, shorter segments of esophagus can tolerate higher levels of radiation than longer segments. The chronic effects of radiation may occur from 6 months to decades after the initial exposure.

The most common chronic complication of radiation therapy is esophageal stricture development due to fibrosis. Esophageal ulcerations, tracheo-esophageal fistulization and esophageal perforation also occur, and are usually due to tumor necrosis. Occasionally, fistulas and ulcerations may involve the aorta, leading to hemorrhage.

Diagnosis

The diagnosis should be suspected in all patients who have a history of esophageal radiation exposure. In the acute setting, upper endoscopy may reveal edema, erythema, erosions, and ulcerations. Chronic radiation esophagitis may involve strictures and chronic ulcers.

Therapy

Treatment of acute effects

Specific treatment for acute esophagitis should address symptom relief and nutritional supplementation. Decreasing the daily radiation dose by 10%, or interrupting therapy temporarily, may help alleviate the acute symptoms of esophagitis. Pain may be controlled using a combination of systemic analgesia (i.e. narcotics) with oral administration of a mixture of viscous lidocaine and mylanta. Proton pump inhibitors or sucralfate may help to decrease any pain exacerbation by gastroesophageal acid reflux.

The role of non-steroidal anti-inflammatory drugs (NSAIDs) is controversial. Some animal models demonstrate prevention of stricture formation, but human studies have not shown such benefit.

Management of chronic complications

Limiting total radiation dose to tolerable levels (less than 60 Gy total) or using oblique or lateral fields to decrease esophageal radiation exposure may limit long-term complications. Strictures may be dilated endoscopically. Patients with strictures refractory to dilation may benefit from semi-solid diets, gastrostomy or other feeding tubes, or esophageal bypass surgery.

Further reading

Baehr PH, McDonald GB. Esophageal infections: risk factors, presentation, diagnosis, and treatment. *Gastroenterology* 1994; 106: 509.

Banerjee S, LaMont JT. Treatment of gastrointestinal infections. *Gastroenterology* 2000; 118: S48–S67.

Buckner FS, Pomeroy C. Cytomegalovirus disease of the gastrointestinal tract in patients without AIDS. *Clin Infect Dis* 1993; 17: 644–656.

Chowhan NM. Injurious effects of radiation on the esophagus. *Am J Gastroenterol* 1990; 85: 115–120.

Eddleston M, Peacock S, Juniper M, *et al.* Severe cytomegalovirus infection in immunocompetent patients. *Clin Infect Dis* 1997; 24: 52.

Gane E, Saliba F, Valdecasas GJ, *et al.* Randomised trial of efficacy and safety of oral ganciclovir in the prevention of cytomegalovirus disease in liver-transplant recipients. The Oral Ganciclovir International Transplantation Study Group. *Lancet* 1997; 350: 1729.

Gumaste W, Dave PB. Ingestion of corrosive substances by adults. *Am J Gastroenterol* 1992; 87: 1.

Kikendall JW. Caustic ingestion injuries. *Gastroenterol Clin North Am* 1991; 20: 847.

Kikendall JW. Pill esophagitis. *J Clin Gastroenterol* 1999; 28: 298–305.

Laine L, Bonacini M. Esophageal disease in Human Immunodeficiency Virus infection. *Arch Intern Med* 1994; 154: 1577–1582.

Levine MS. Drug-induced disorders of the esophagus. *Abdom Imaging* 1999; 24: 3–8.

Ramanathan J, Rammouni M, Baran Jr J, *et al.* Herpes Simplex Virus esophagitis in the immunocompetent host: An overview. *Am J Gastroenterol* 2000; 95:2171–2176.

Whitley RJ, Jacobson MA, Friedberg DN, *et al.* Guidelines for the treatment of cytomegalovirus diseases in patients with AIDS in the era of potent antiretroviral therapy: Recommendations of an international panel. *Arch Intern Med* 1998; 158: 957.

Wilcox CM, Straub RF, Schwartz DA. Cytomegalovirus esophagitis in AIDS: A prospective evaluation of clinical response to ganciclovir therapy, relapse rate and long-term outcome. *Am J Med* 1995; 98: 169.

Chapter 3

Barrett's Esophagus

Michelle Beilstein and Debra G. Silberg

CHAPTER OUTLINE

Earlier definitions have restricted Barrett's esophagus to intestinal metaplasia 3 cm or more above the squamocolumnar junction, "long-segment Barrett's". After the discovery of mucosa rich in goblet cells, a marker of intestinal metaplasia, at the gastroesophageal junction, the definition of Barrett's esophagus was extended to include this variant known as "short-segment Barrett's". Thus, the incidence of Barrett's esophagus has increased over time as currently the definition of Barrett's esophagus includes all intestinal metaplasia above the gastroesophageal junction. The epidemiology of short-segment versus long-segment Barrett's esophagus is currently unfolding. Of note, the incidence of Barrett's esophagus has also increased in conjunction with an increase in the frequency of upper endoscopy.

Epidemiology

Barrett's esophagus, intestinal metaplasia of the esophagus, is a premalignant condition of the esophagus leading to esophageal adenocarcinoma. It has been identified in up to 20% of patients undergoing endoscopy for gastroesophageal reflux symptoms and is estimated to occur in at least 700 000 adults in the US. These figures are evolving as the definition of Barrett's esophagus has changed over time.

Risk factors and pathophysiology

Many risk factors have been evaluated with respect to Barrett's esophagus. Those with a positive association are listed in Box 3.1.

Barrett's esophagus typically occurs in Caucasian men aged 40 to 63 years of age. Although the risk of Barrett's esophagus increases with age, it can occur in patients of all ages. Many pediatric cases of Barrett's esophagus

Box 3.1 Risk factors associated with Barrett's esophagus

Caucasian men.
Age over 50 years.
Duration of reflux symptoms for more than 5 years.
Development of reflux symptoms at an early age.
Nocturnal reflux symptoms.
Obesity.
Possibly tobacco and/or ethanol.
Hiatal hernia.
Abnormal lower esophageal sphincter pressure.
Abnormal 24-hour pH study.

have been reported in the literature. The male to female ratio is estimated at 1.5:1 for benign Barrett's esophagus and up to 3.1:1 for esophageal adenocarcinoma. Barrett's esophagus occurs fourteen times more commonly in whites than in African Americans and is even more uncommon in the Asian population. Hispanics in North and South America have a similar risk of Barrett's esophagus to Caucasians.

Other risk factors for Barrett's esophagus include a long duration of GERD symptoms, development of reflux at an early age, increased severity of nocturnal reflux symptoms and obesity. However, patients with Barrett's esophagus are generally indistinguishable from those with GERD who do not have Barrett's esophagus. It is controversial whether tobacco and/or ethanol intake predispose patients to Barrett's esophagus, but these activities do increase reflux symptoms. Several studies have suggested that infection with the cag A strain of *Helicobacter pylori* may protect against the development of Barrett's esophagus and the progression to dysplasia and adenocarcinoma.

Why some patients with reflux get Barrett's esophagus while others do not is currently not understood. The complete pathophysiology of Barrett's esophagus remains to be elucidated. Studies have shown that manometrically determined abnormal lower esophageal sphincter pressure, abnormal acid exposure on a 24-hour pH study, or presence of a hiatal hernia occur in greater than 60% of patients with short- or long-segment Barrett's esophagus. These figures increase to over 80% if only patients with long-segment Barrett's esophagus are included.

Hydrochloric acid, pepsin, and trypsin are believed to be the most harmful substances in the gastric refluxate and are known to cause severe esophagitis. Controversy exists over the role of bile reflux leading to Barrett's esophagus. Some have found a direct correlation with complicated GERD (esophagitis and Barrett's esophagus) with higher exposure to acid and bile reflux. Interestingly, exposure to bile salts or acid enhances esophageal epithelial cell proliferation, while effective therapy with acid-suppressive agents inhibits esophageal epithelial cell proliferation favoring differentiation of esophageal epithelial cells. Yet, clinical studies show no increased risk of either long- or short-segment Barrett's esophagus in patients with gastric surgery for peptic ulcer disease. Rat models have been used to show that the presence of acid protects rodents from developing adenocarcinoma secondary to bile and carcinogen exposure. In time such controversies will be sorted out as our understanding of the pathophysiology of Barrett's esophagus improves.

Diagnosis

Recent data have revealed that only 5% of patients with esophageal adenocarcinoma, likely arising from Barrett's esophagus, were diagnosed with Barrett's esophagus prior to the diagnosis of the esophageal adenocarcinoma. These data support routine screening programs for patients at risk for Barrett's esophagus. Screening should be focused on those with the greatest risk factors as listed in Box 3.1. This includes white men who are 50 years of age or older, with nocturnal or long-standing reflux symptoms (symptoms for greater than 5 years), or with reflux symptoms that do not abate with medical therapy, or who are obese. Unfortunately, this type of screening program is unlikely to detect all patients with Barrett's esophagus because many patients are asymptomatic. How best to diagnosis all patients at risk is currently under study.

The only effective form of screening for Barrett's esophagus is by upper endoscopy with biopsy. The classical finding of Barrett's esophagus at endoscopy is salmon-pink tongues of tissue arising from and extending proximal to the squamocolumnar junction (Figure 3.1A). Some studies have used various vital stains to help in the recognition of Barrett's esophagus. Such stains include Lugol's iodine, toluidine blue, indigo carmine, and methylene blue. Most endoscopists do not use these stains as their use has not been shown to improve the recognition of Barrett's esophagus. Biopsies of suspicious areas must reveal intestinal metaplasia with histological evidence of goblet cells (Figure 3.1B). Goblet cells are specialized mucin-producing cells found only

in the small and large intestinal mucosa and are readily seen on histology with an alcian blue stain. At the time of screening any nodular, ulcerated lesions should be biopsied as many patients are diagnosed with esophageal adenocarcinoma at the index endoscopy for Barrett's esophagus. Once the diagnosis of Barrett's esophagus is made, patients should be treated with acid suppression and enrolled in a surveillance program to detect dysplasia or curable esophageal adenocarcinoma.

Esophageal adenocarcinoma from Barrett's

Esophageal adenocarcinoma has increased tenfold over that past few decades and is thought to arise from Barrett's esophagus. No other cancer has increased faster with respect to incidence, especially among white males. Recent publications have shown that the same risk factors for Barrett's esophagus; longer duration of GERD symptoms, development of reflux at an early age, and increased severity

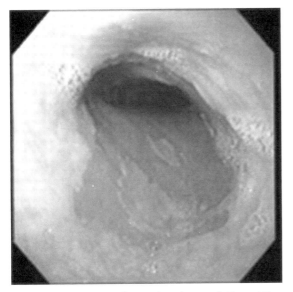
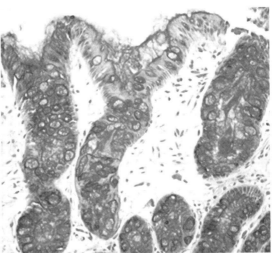

Figure 3.1 A. Endoscopic view of Barrett's esophagus. B. Histology of Barrett's esophagus, highlighting goblet cells with alcian blue staining, × 200. (See p. xvii for color)

of nocturnal reflux symptoms, are also associated with an increase risk of developing adenocarcinoma of the esophagus. Earlier and smaller studies on the risk of Barrett's esophagus developing into esophageal adenocarcinoma may have overestimated this risk through publication bias. However, more recent studies have estimated the risk of developing adenocarcinoma from Barrett's esophagus to be about 0.4% to 0.5% per patient years of follow-up. Patients with short-segment Barrett's esophagus are also at risk of developing esophageal adenocarcinoma, but this risk is believed to be even lower than those with longer segments of Barrett's esophagus.

It is believed that Barrett's esophagus progresses in a step-wise fashion from metaplasia to low-grade dysplasia to high-grade dysplasia (HGD) to adenocarcinoma. Research efforts have focused on understanding the metaplasia–dysplasia–carcinoma sequence. One area of interest is the development of markers to diagnose and assess cancer risk in patients with Barrett's esophagus. The most promising genetic abnormalities studied to date include tumor suppressors, such as p53, p16 and adenomatous polyposis coli (APC) mutations, and aneuploidy (increased DNA content). The p53 mutation is one of the most common somatic genetic mutations in human cancers and the most widely studied. When p53 is mutated, cells with damaged DNA can replicate, leading to abnormal cells with increased DNA content. Abnormal p53 expression rarely occurs in Barrett's esophagus without dysplasia, but inactivation of p53 occurs in 60% of patients with HGD and in up to 95% of patients with esophageal adenocarcinoma. Both p16 and APC are tumor suppressor genes associated with colon cancer. Loss of p16 or APC is rarely seen in Barrett's metaplasia without dysplasia, but may be present in Barrett's metaplasia with dysplasia and esophageal adenocarcinomas. Flow cytometric studies have been used to identify cell populations with abnormal DNA content in Barrett's esophagus. There is a linear

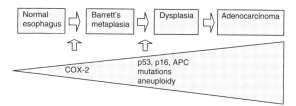

Figure 3.2 Diagram of the common changes in the progression to adenocarcinoma.

increase in aneuploid populations in the progression from Barrett's without dysplasia to Barrett's with dysplasia and adenocarcinoma (Figure 3.2).

Studies have shown that the 5-year survival of patients with esophageal adenocarcinoma is only 17% after surgical resection and less than 1% for unresectable tumors. Unfortunately, in most patients, esophageal adenocarcinoma is discovered at an unresectable stage lending to a poor prognosis. Patients who are elderly are often poor surgical candidates and esophagectomy carries its own risks of morbidity and mortality. The surgical literature reports a 30% to 70% rate of invasive cancer in esophagectomy specimens removed for HGD. Thus, patients with HGD, who are good surgical candidates, should undergo esophagectomy to remove areas of undiagnosed adenocarcinoma or to avoid the development of esophageal adenocarcinoma. Operative mortality rates are directly related to the number of esophagectomies that the particular surgeon who is operating has performed in the past. One study showed a mortality rate of 3% to 4.2% in a high-volume center versus 12.2% to 13.3% in a low-volume center. Thus, esophagectomy for HGD or adenocarcinoma should be undertaken at a high-volume center to decrease the risk of operative mortality.

Surveillance

At present it is impossible to know which patients will progress from Barrett's esophagus to esophageal adenocarcinoma. Thus, surveillance programs have been in place for some time to identify patients at risk for progressing from metaplasia to dysplasia to adenocarcinoma (Figure 3.3). It has been recommended that patients undergo endoscopy with four quadrant biopsies at 2 cm intervals in all abnormal-appearing tissue which might contain Barrett's esophagus. This is most properly done with jumbo biopsy forceps using a therapeutic endoscope with a turn and suction technique to increase the yield of tissue. Abnormalities such as nodules, erosions, or luminal irregularities should be biopsied first to avoid obscuring them with blood from other biopsy sites. Such surveillance should occur only after inflammation from GERD is controlled with appropriate anti-secretory therapy, i.e. proton pump inhibitors.

Without knowing the actual risk of developing esophageal adenocarcinoma from Barrett's esophagus it is difficult to determine the most cost-effective method to survey these patients. Thus, the interval for surveillance endoscopy is evolving. Current recommendations include endoscopy with appropriate biopsies every year for 2 initial years. If these endoscopies are negative for dysplasia then the interval can be expanded to every 2 to 3 years. However, for patients with low-grade dysplasia, the recommendation is to do endoscopy with surveillance biopsy every 6 months for 1 year followed by annual endoscopy with surveillance biopsy if there is no progression of dysplasia. Controversy exists over the follow-up of patients with HGD. Recent data suggest a 3.7-fold increase in the risk of esophageal cancer in patients with diffuse HGD versus patients with focal HGD. The gold standard for therapy in patients with HGD remains esophagectomy, but given the morbidity and mortality of esophagectomy, patients with focal

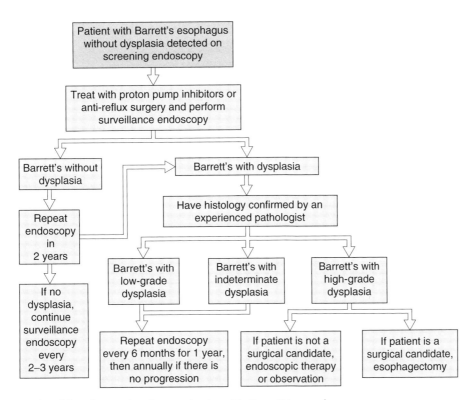

Figure 3.3 Algorithm for evaluating patients with Barrett's esophagus.

HGD may be candidates for continued surveillance for adenocarcinoma and endoscopic therapies. There is still a risk of transformation from HGD to esophageal adenocarcinoma and this risk should be discussed thoroughly with patients wishing to undergo such surveillance instead of proceeding to esophagectomy. These patients should also be evaluated by endoscopic ultrasound to detect unsuspected adenocarcinoma with submucosal invasion and lymph-node involvement. Patients with diffuse HGD who are young and good surgical candidates should undergo esophagectomy. Patients who are poor surgical candidates, who refuse esophagectomy, or who desire continued surveillence should undergo repeat endoscopy with biopsies within 1 month of initial diagnosis of HGD with biopsies taken at 1 cm intervals instead of 2 cm to assess a larger surface area for adenocarcinoma. In these patients, surveillance should be continued every 3 months as long as the patient remains a candidate for therapy.

Surveillance intervals have not been subjected to randomized controlled trials and are based on our limited understanding of the metaplasia–dysplasia–adenocarcinoma sequence that can progress in Barrett's esophagus. A recent cost analysis study using an epidemiological model and an annual cancer risk of 0.4% annually revealed surveillance for Barrett's esophagus without dysplasia every 5 years to be most cost effective. To substantiate these intervals a large number of patients would need to be enrolled in a multicenter-type trial.

Reports in the literature suggest that most esophageal adenocarcinomas are not found in patients undergoing surveillance and those patients diagnosed with esophageal adenocarcinoma do not have a precancerous diagnosis of Barrett's esophagus. However, esophageal adenocarcinomas found in surveillance programs tend to be diagnosed at earlier stages than those presenting with symptoms outside a surveillance program. Of note, studies of resected esophageal specimens have shown that HGD and early esophageal adenocarcinoma in Barrett's esophagus can occur in the absence of endoscopic abnormalities.

The diagnosis of dysplasia is not always clear because there can be differences in the interpretation of biopsies by individual pathologists. This leads to inter-observer variability further complicating diagnosis, surveillance, and treatment strategy. Thus, biopsies read as having dysplasia should be re-evaluated by another experienced pathologist.

Treatment (Table 3.1)

Medical therapy

Medical therapy with a proton pump inhibitor to suppress acid, should be the first intervention for Barrett's esophagus treatment. It has been determined that an increase in quantity of acid reflux is the single most characteristic feature of patients with Barrett's esophagus. In addition, proton pump inhibitors have been shown to decrease both acid and bile reflux, which may be synergistic in causing mucosal damage. Symptoms do not predict the quality of acid control in patients taking proton pump inhibitors. Many patients with Barrett's esophagus on medical therapy exhibit no symptoms; however, follow-up 24-hour pH studies reveal periods of uncontrolled acid reflux, even on high doses of proton pump inhibitors. It is, however, not feasible to test a 24-hour pH on all patients with Barrett's esophagus who are taking a proton pump inhibitor. Patients with Barrett's esophagus appear to be less symptomatic to acid reflux than patients with uncomplicated GERD. Interestingly, there are some patients who are completely asymptomatic without any anti-secretory therapy. Therapy with high doses of proton pump inhibitors leads to only rare cases of regression of Barrett's esophagus. Such therapy has not yet been proven

Table 3.1 Treatment modalities

Therapy	Pros and Cons
Medical therapy with proton pump inhibitor	First line of therapy for acid suppression. May not be effective in all patients, even with relief of symptoms. Not proven to cause regression or stop progression of Barrett's esophagus.
Anti-reflux surgery	Restores lower esophageal sphincter function, abolishes reflux. 85% effective in immediate post-operative period. Long-term results vary. Risks include surgical mortality, dysphagia, inability to belch and vomit. Not proven to cause regression or stop progression of Barrett's esophagus, may be more difficult to perform surveillance.
Endoscopic therapy	Alternative for non-surgical candidates with dysplasia or adenocarcinoma (not proven effective). Ablative therapy may result in trapped Barrett's mucosa under squamous epithelium. Complications include: photodynamic therapy: skin phototoxicity, strictures, dysphagia endoscopic mucosal resection: dysphagia, bleeding, perforation thermal ablative therapy: dysphagia, perforation, chest pain.

effective in the prevention of esophageal adenocarcinoma. Studies have shown that effective intra-esophageal acid suppression in patients with Barrett's esophagus favors differentiation and decreases proliferation of esophageal mucosal cells.

Anti-reflux surgery

The Nissen fundoplication is the most commonly used type of anti-reflux operation and can often be done laparoscopically. The indications for anti-reflux surgery are listed in Box 3.2. Fundoplication should be considered in patients with minimal surgical risk, who do not want to take, are not compliant with, or have not had sufficient acid control with proton pump inhibitors. Anti-reflux surgery is believed to be effective by restoring the lower esophageal sphincter function and abolishing

Box 3.2 Indications for anti-reflux surgery

Symptoms of GERD uncontrolled with medical therapy: proton pump inhibitors.
The need for lifelong medical therapy.
Non-compliance by the patient with medical therapy.
Reflux-induced aspiration pneumonia.
Failure of medical therapy to control extra-intestinal manifestations of reflux: laryngitis or asthma.

reflux of gastric contents into the esophagus. Studies have shown greater efficacy of anti-reflux surgical procedures over medical therapy with H_2-receptor antagonists. But these medications are less effective than the currently available proton pump inhibitors. Anti-reflux surgery is reported to be 85% effective in relieving symptoms in the immediate post-operative period; however long-term follow-up indicates that symptoms recur in some of these patients secondary to breakdown of the operation or failure of the operation to control symptoms. A recent randomized controlled trial on the long-term outcome of medical and surgical therapies for GERD revealed that up to 62% of patients who underwent anti-reflux surgery regularly used anti-reflux medications (proton pump inhibitors, H_2-receptor blockers, or prokinetic agents) post-operatively. Patients with symptoms after fundoplication, thought to be due to reflux, should have a 24-hour pH study to determine whether the symptoms are due to acid reflux.

Collective data from many studies looking at the results of anti-reflux therapy for Barrett's esophagus reveal no change in histology in 74% of patients, regression in 17% of patients, and progression in 9% of patients. After fundoplication endoscopic surveillance may be more difficult because it is possible that a portion of the esophagus may be included in the wrap. Many institutions report cases of esophageal adenocarcinoma in patients with Barrett's esophagus who have undergone anti-reflux operations. Interestingly, one study reported occurrences of esophageal cancer in only the first 39 months after anti-reflux surgery.

Morbidity rates of anti-reflux surgery are estimated to be 8%. The most common complications of anti-reflux surgery are dysphagia and the inability to belch or vomit. The mortality rate from anti-reflux surgery is less than 1%. One long-term follow-up study reported a significant decrease in survival in surgically treated patients compared to medically treated patients secondary to deaths due to heart disease.

Endoscopic therapy

Recently there have been efforts to find endoscopic approaches to ablate the metaplastic or dysplastic epithelium of Barrett's esoph-agus. Such approaches include photodynamic therapy and endoscopic mucosal resection for the treatment of patients with HGD or superficial esophageal adenocarcinoma. Patients appropriate for these therapies are not surgical candidates usually because of co-morbid illnesses. Thermal ablative therapies have been used to treat Barrett's esophagus with or without low-grade dysplasia. These ablative techniques attempt to destroy the metaplastic mucosa and promote the regrowth of squamous epithelium with the hopes of decreasing the risk of cancer. To date, a decrease in cancer risk has not been demonstrated with any of these methods. Endoscopic therapies are not standard-of-care at this time and should only be used in patients with dysplasia or adenocarcinoma who are not deemed surgical candidates, or who are part of a clinical research study.

Photodynamic therapy (PDT)

To perform PDT a photosensitizer, porfimer sodium in the US, is given intravenously to patients 2 days prior to the scheduled endoscopic treatment. For unclear reasons, this agent has a predilection for neoplastic tissue and the delay of 2 days allows the photosensitizer to reach an optimal level within the neoplastic tissue compared to normal tissue. During endoscopy a red light is shone on the segment of Barrett's epithelium activating the photosensitizer. Once activated, the photosensitizer turns oxygen molecules into highly reactive singlet oxygen which causes cell death of the dysplastic and neoplastic tissue. Endoscopic therapy is followed by high-dose acid suppression allowing the squamous mucosa to regenerate and replace the Barrett's esophagus tissue.

Studies have shown HGD response rates of 88% to 100%. Unfortunately, in 4% to 40% of patients the squamous mucosa can overgrow areas of the mucosa containing Barrett's esophagus leading to pockets of trapped

Barrett's metaplasia. One study revealed that despite histological improvement in dysplasia, genetic abnormalities, such as p53 mutations and aneuploidy, persist after PDT. Thus, these patients still have the genetic alterations thought to be involved in the progression from dysplasia to adenocarcinoma. In fact the literature reports one patient who underwent PDT for HGD and was later diagnosed with adenocarcinoma underlying normal squamous mucosa.

The complications of photodynamic therapy include severe skin phototoxicity (patients must not be exposed to intense light exposure for 30 to 90 days after therapy), esophageal strictures, chest pain, dysphagia, and small unilateral or bilateral pleural effusions. Because of the possibility of severe complications, such as stricture, this therapy should not be used in Barrett's esophagus without dysplasia.

Endoscopic mucosal resection (EMR)

Once an area of HGD or superficial adenocarcinoma is detected on routine biopsy EMR can be scheduled if the patient is not a surgical candidate. During endoscopy a saline and epinephrine mixture is injected into the submucosal layer detaching the lesion from the deeper mucosal layers by lifting the lesion. The raised area is then either resected using a snare or a variceal ligating device. The tissue that is removed is sent for histological evaluation to determine the depth of penetration of the lesion, the size of the lesion, and the margins of resection. This is a valuable tool for resecting localized HGD or superficial, esophageal adenocarcinoma, and it can also aid in the diagnosis of suspicious lesions. Complications of EMR include dysphagia, bleeding, and esophageal perforation. More recent data have shown that EMR followed by photodynamic therapy can be safe and possibly more effective than either therapy alone.

Thermal ablative therapy

Thermal ablative therapies with such devices as the argon plasma coagulator or multipolar electrocautery (MPEC) devices have been used in an attempt to ablate the mucosa of Barrett's esophagus without dysplasia or with low-grade dysplasia. The goal to this therapy is the ablation of Barrett's esophagus followed by high-dose acid suppression to allow normal esophageal squamous tissue to overgrow and replace the Barrett's esophagus segment. Studies have shown these techniques to be effective in 61% to 98% of patients. Unfortunately, thermal ablation therapy may lead to squamous epithelium with trapped Barrett's esophagus below or regrowth of the Barrett's metaplasia at an increased length. Other complications have included chest pain, dysphagia, esophageal perforation, and death.

Chemoprevention

Studies have shown a decreased incidence of esophageal adenocarcinoma in patients who take aspirin or NSAIDs; the latter are COX inhibitors (cyclooxygenase-enzyme inhibitors). The cyclooxygenase enzymes convert arachadonic acid to inflammatory mediators with an associated decrease in cell–cell adhesion and programed cell death, and an increase in angiogenesis and proliferation. The expression of COX-2 increases in the progression from Barrett's metaplasia to dysplasia and to adenocarcinoma (Figure 3.2). One group has shown an increase in COX-2 expression in response to pulses of acid or bile salts in an *ex vivo* esophageal organ culture model. A selective COX-2 inhibitor attenuated the effect of acid and bile salts on the cells. This, and other experiments, have laid the foundation for ongoing clinical studies using COX-2 inhibitors as chemopreventive agents in patients with Barrett's esophagus.

Further reading

Beilstein M, Silberg D. Cellular and molecular mechanisms responsible for progression of Barrett's metaplasia to esophageal adenocarcinoma. *Gastroenterol Clin N Am* 2002; 31: 461–479.

Buttar NS, Wang KK, Sebo TJ, *et al*. Extent of high-grade dysplasia in Barrett's esophagus correlated with risk of adenocarcinoma. *Gastroenterology* 2001; 120: 1630–1639.

DeMeester SR, DeMeester TR. The diagnosis and management of Barrett's esophagus. *Advances in Surgery* 1999; 33: 29–68.

Dulai GS, Guha S, Kahn KL, *et al*. Preoperative prevalence of Barrett's esophagus in esophageal adenocarcinoma: a systematic review. *Gastroenterology*, 2002; 122: 26–33.

Lagergren J, Bergstrom R, Lindgren A, *et al*. Symptomatic gastroesophageal reflux as a risk factor for esophageal adenocarcinoma. *New Engl J Med* 1999; 340: 825–831.

Nandurkar S, Talley NJ. Barrett's esophagus: the long and short of it. *Am J Gastroenterol* 1999; 94: 30–40.

Ouatu-Lascar R, Fitzgerald RC, Triadafilopoulos G. Differentiation and proliferation in Barrett's esophagus and the effects of acid suppression. *Gastroenterology* 1999; 117: 327–335.

Provenzale D, Schmitt C, Wong JB. Barrett's esophagus: a new look at surveillance based on emerging estimates of cancer risk. *Am J Gastroenterol* 1999; 94: 2043–2053.

Reynolds JC, Waronker M, Pacquing MS, *et al*. Barrett's esophagus: reducing the risk of progression to adenocarcinoma. *Gastroenterol Clin N Am* 1999; 28: 917–945.

Sampliner MD. Practice Guidelines: updated guidelines for the diagnosis, surveillance, and therapy of Barrett's esophagus. *Am J Gastroenterol* 2002; 97: 1888–1895.

Schulz H, Miehlke S, Antos D, *et al*. Ablation of Barrett's epithelium by endoscopic argon plasma coagulation in combination with high-dose omeprazole. *Gastrointest Endosc* 2000; 6: 659–663.

Scotiniotis IA, Kochman ML, Lewis JD, *et al*. Accuracy of EUS in the evaluation of Barrett's esophagus and high-grade dysplasia or intramucosal carcinoma. *Gastrointest Endosc* 2001; 54: 689–696.

Spechler SJ, Lee E, Ahnen D, *et al*. Long-term outcome of medical and surgical therapies for gastroesophageal reflux disease: follow-up of randomized controlled trial. *JAMA* 2001; 285: 2331–2338.

Spechler SJ. Barrett's esophagus. *New Engl J Med* 2002; 346: 836–842.

Wang KK, Sampliner RE. Mucosal ablation therapy of Barrett's esophagus. *Mayo Clin Proc* 2001; 76: 433–437.

Chapter 4

Esophageal Motility Disorders

Yu-Xiao Yang and David A. Katzka

CHAPTER OUTLINE

Introduction

The esophagus is a muscular tube with two sphincters at the ends, acting as a conduit for the transport of food from the oral cavity to the stomach. The proper function of the esophagus relies on the anatomic and physiologic specialization of the esophageal muscle and nervous system. When the neuromuscular apparatus of these structures fails to properly function, a motility disorder ensues. Motility disorders of the esophagus encompass a wide spectrum of entities characterized by symptoms suspected of being esophageal in origin (e.g., chest pain, dysphagia) and abnormal esophageal motility patterns. To understand the pathophysiology of esophageal motility disorders, it is important to review the normal anatomy of the esophagus and its normal physiology.

Anatomy

The muscularis propria of the esophagus is responsible for carrying out the organ's motor function. The esophageal wall comprises inner circular and outer longitudinal layers of muscle. Unlike the rest of the intestinal tract, no serosa is found over the esophagus. Generally, the upper 5% to 33% is composed of skeletal muscle, and the distal 66% is composed of smooth muscle. At the junction is a mixture of both types. Proximally, the esophagus begins where the inferior pharyngeal constrictor merges with the cricopharyngeus, an area of skeletal muscle known functionally as the upper esophageal sphincter (UES). The UES is contracted at rest and thereby creates a high-pressure zone that prevents both inspired air from entering the esophagus, and esophageal content from entering the oropharynx and larynx. The esophageal body lies within the posterior mediastinum behind the trachea and left mainstem bronchus and swings leftward to pass behind the heart and in front of the aorta. Within the diaphragmatic hiatus the esophageal body ends in a 2- to 4-cm length of asymmetrically thickened circular smooth muscle known as the lower esophageal sphincter (LES). The phrenoesophageal ligament, which originates from the diaphragm's transversalis fascia and inserts on the lower esophagus, contributes to fixation of the LES within the diaphragmatic hiatus. This positioning is beneficial because it enables diaphragmatic contractions to assist the LES in maintenance of a high-pressure zone during exercise. The LES is contracted at rest, creating a high-pressure zone that prevents gastric contents from entering the esophagus. During swallowing, the LES relaxes to permit the swallowed bolus to be pushed by peristalsis from the esophagus into the stomach.

Both parasympathetic and sympathetic nerves innervate the esophageal wall; the parasympathetics regulate peristalsis through the vagus nerve. Medullary vagal postganglionic efferent nerves terminate directly on the motor endplate of the skeletal muscle of the upper esophagus, whereas vagal preganglionic efferent nerves to the smooth muscle of the distal esophagus terminate on neurons within Auerbach's (myenteric) plexus, located between the circular and longitudinal muscle layers. A second neuronal sensory network, Meissner's plexus, located within the submucosa, is the site of afferent impulses arising within the esophageal wall. These are transmitted to the central nervous system through both vagal parasympathetic and thoracic sympathetic nerves.

Physiology of swallowing

Swallowing involves a complex coordination of the oropharyngeal and esophageal neuromuscular components. The initial phase of swallowing is the oral phase. In this phase, a food bolus is transferred posteriorly into the pharynx when the tongue pushes against the palate sequentially in an anterior-to-posterior order. Since the muscle of the oropharynx is striated, this phase of swallowing in under central nervous system control. During the next phase, the pharyngeal phase, swallowing is not under conscious control. In addition, the swallowing center and respiratory center of the medulla are involved in this phase. The coordination between these two centers ensures the closure of UES during respiration and closure of the larynx and nasopharynx during swallowing. The respiration is inhibited during this phase. The UES relaxes to allow passage of the food bolus. The third phase of swallowing is the esophageal phase, in which peristalsis takes place. In this phase, the longitudinal muscle contracts and shortens the esophagus. The circular smooth muscle contracts to generate primary, secondary or non-peristaltic tertiary contraction.

Oropharyngeal dysphagia

Oropharyngeal dysphagia is an important problem in our aging population. Nearly one third of all stroke patients develop oropharyngeal dysphagia. Up to 60% of nursing-home occupants have feeding difficulties, a significant proportion of whom have oropharyngeal dysphagia. There are a plethora of causes of oropharyngeal dysphagia (Table 4.1). These causes can be categorized into six groups: structural, neurological, iatrogenic, infectious, myopathic, and drug or metabolic causes. Oropharyngeal dysphagia is strongly associated with head injuries, Parkinson's disease, and Alzheimer's disease, and it carries a high morbidity, mortality, and medical cost. Oropharyngeal dysphagia differs from esophageal dysphagia in several important aspects. First, oropharyngeal dysphagia carries a high risk of aspiration and its life-threatening sequelae. Second, while primary esophageal diseases usually cause esophageal dysphagia, oropharyngeal dysphagia is most commonly due to neurogenic or myogenic diseases in which dysphagia is frequently a part of a wider neurological syndrome.

Clinical assessment of oropharyngeal dysphagia

A careful history may help distinguish oropharyngeal dysphagia from esophageal dysphagia or globus sensation. Typical symptoms in patients with oropharyngeal dysphagia include drooling, spillage of food because of weakness in facial or labial muscles, xeros-

tomia or sialorrhea, difficulty in initiating swallowing, piecemeal swallows, dysarthria, sensation of food stuck in the neck, postnasal regurgitation, coughing or choking during meals, a need for repeated swallows to clear food or liquid from the pharynx, and dysphonia. Patients with persistent sore throat or pain when swallowing may have underlying malignancy or inflammatory/infectious process. Delayed regurgitation of food may suggest the presence of a pharyngeal diverticulum. Solid-food predominant dysphagia is more consistent with a structural lesion such as stenosis, web, or tumor.

The onset, duration, and associated symptoms may also be helpful in ascertaining the underlying cause of the oropharyngeal dysphagia. Progressive dysphagia associated with weight loss may suggest underlying malignancy. A sudden onset of oropharyngeal dysphagia in combination with other neurologic deficits is more consistent with a stroke. Progressive dysphagia in combination with widespread neuromuscular symptoms is present in motor neuron disease and myopathies. Tremor and ataxia suggest Parkinson's disease. A careful medication history is necessary to exclude drug-related causes of oropharyngeal dysphagia. A complete physical examination including a thorough neurological examination is mandatory in light of the multisystemic nature of the symptom complex often encountered in patients with oropharyngeal dysphagia.

Diagnostic evaluation

The evaluation of patients with suspected oropharyngeal dysphagia includes video-esophagram, fiberoptic endoscopic evaluation of swallowing (FEES), and manometry. The videoesophagram acquires dedicated lateral and anteroposterior views of the oral and pharyngeal phases of the swallow and

Table 4.1 Causes of oropharyngeal dysphagia (adapted with permission from Cook IJ, Kahrilas PJ. AGA: Technical review – management of oropharyngeal dysphagia. *Gastroenterology* 1999; 116: 455)

Structural causes	Cricopharyngeal bar Zenker's diverticulum Cervical webs Oropharyngeal tumors Osteophytes Congenital (cleft palate, diverticula, etc.)
Neurological causes	Brain tumors Head trauma Stroke Cerebral palsy Guillain-Barré syndrome Huntington's disease Multiple sclerosis Polio Postpolio syndrome Tardive dyskinesia Metabolic encephalopathies Amyotrophic lateral sclerosis Parkinson's disease Dementia
Myopathic causes	Connective tissue disease Dermatomyositis Myasthenia gravis Myotonic dystrophy Oculopharyngeal dystrophy Polymyositis Sarcoidosis Paraneoplastic syndrome
Drug or metabolic causes	Amyloidosis Cushing's syndrome Thyrotoxicosis Wilson's disease
Infectious causes	Diptheria Botulism Lyme disease Syphilis Mucositis (e.g. herpes, cytomegalovirus, candida)
Iatrogenic causes	Radiation Surgical complications Corrosive injury (e.g., pill-induced, caustic) Medication side effects (e.g., neuroleptics, chemotherapy)

permits standard and slow motion replay of the swallow. This technique allows appreciation of the mechanics and severity of the swallow dysfunction. One of the most important pieces of information provided by videoesophagram is the presence, timing and severity of aspiration. Other abnormalities identifiable by this technique include the absence of or delayed pharyngeal swallow response, impaired pharyngeal clearance of contrast, and velopharyngeal competence in the presence of aspiration. It also gives good anatomic definition of the UES, laryngeal and basilar tongue structures. Patients with oropharyngeal dysphagia may also be identified by videoesophagram for significantly increased risk for aspiration pneumonia.

Fiberoptic nasoendoscopy is less well suited for the assessment of swallowing mechanics than videoesophagram, but it is an ideal method for identifying and biopsying mucosal abnormalities. Its sensitivity in identifying glottic and pharyngeal cancer is far superior to esophagogastroduodenoscopy. Therefore, it is mandatory in all cases in which malignancy is suspected. Fiberoptic endoscopic evaluation of swallowing (FEES) is also a useful technique in identifying evidence of aspiration. It can be performed unassisted by a speech pathologist with standard fiberoptic instrumentation, and is rapidly becoming the procedure of choice for the evaluation of swallowing function in many clinical settings, including the intensive care unit, with stroke patients, and with patients who have chronic neuromuscular disorders.

On the other hand, pharyngeal manometry can quantify pharyngeal deglutitive pressure and detect failure of UES relaxation and discoordination of pharyngeal contraction. However, it is technically demanding and prone to interference due to unpredictable structural movement during the pharyngeal swallow phase. Therefore, its clinical use is limited compared to videoesophagram and FEES. It may, however, sometimes supply complementary information.

Management of oropharyngeal dysphagia

The first step in the management of oropharyngeal dysphagia is to determine the risk of aspiration pneumonia. The second step is to identify and treat the underlying cause. It important to remember that silent aspiration occurs in many of these patients, and clinical determination of aspiration underestimates the risk of aspiration pneumonia by 50% compared to videoesophagram. Videoesophagram evaluation may also provide information regarding the potential benefit of gastrostomy feeding in reducing the risk of aspiration. The fourth step is the institution of therapies specific for the swallowing dysfunction. These include dietary modification, swallowing therapy, and/or surgery. Simple dietary modification can reduce the risk of aspiration pneumonia. Swallowing therapy, guided by videoesophagram findings, aims to strengthen the weak pharyngeal muscle groups and improve the coordination and mechanics of pharyngeal swallowing. Cricopharyngeal myotomy for cricopharyngeal disorders may be effective where the UES is hypertensive or poorly compliant. Recently, botulinum toxin injections of the UES have also been used. However, its role for neuromyogenic oropharyngeal dysphagia is unclear. In patients who demonstrate aspiration of oral secretions as a cause of recurrent pneumonias, surgical procedures aimed at eliminating oral secretions may be indicated (e.g. epiglottoplasty, partial or total cricoid excision, laryngeal suspension, vocal-fold medialization, glottic closure, laryngotracheal diversion, or laryngectomy).

Globus sensation

Epidemiology

Globus is an extremely common sensation of fullness in the back of the throat. About 45% of healthy subjects in one study have experienced it at least once, usually during emotional events. Persistent or recurrent globus sensation also occurs in many patients, accounting for about 4% of the new patients seen in general otolaryngology clinics.

Etiology

In contrast to oropharyngeal dysphagia, patients with globus sensation do not have food-bolus-transport dysfunctions. It is associated with a number of cervical, pharyngeal, and esophageal disorders (Box 4.1). However, the etiology of globus sensation is poorly understood.

Gastroesophageal reflux disease has been linked with globus sensation. Some clinical studies have shown that patients with globus sensation are more likely to have abnormal pH studies and to have symptoms of reflux than normal controls. It has also been speculated that

Box 4.1 Diseases associated with globus sensation (adapted from Moser G, *et al. Arch Intern Med* 1998;158(12):1365-1373).

GERD
Goiters
Post-uvulopalatoplasty
Achalasia
Carcinoma of the base of the tongue
Hyperplastic tonsils
Hypertensive upper esophageal sphincter
Postcricoid web
Paraesophageal mass
Hiatal hernia

distal esophageal acid exposure in GERD may induce UES contraction, leading to globus sensation. However, this theory has not been proven in clinical studies. Overall, the available evidence suggests that GERD may play a role in the pathogenesis of globus sensation.

Upper esophageal sphincter abnormality has also been suggested as a cause of globus sensation based on the observation in some studies that hypertensive UES is more common among patients with globus sensation than controls. Furthermore, there appears to be an increased prevalence of psychiatric disorders, such as somatization, anxiety disorder, and depression, in patients with globus sensation than in controls.

Clinical manifestation

Patients usually describe a persistent or intermittent sensation of a lump or foreign body in the throat. These sensations typically occur between meals. Dysphagia and odynophagia are usually absent. The sensation is often induced by states of fear, tension, anger, or mental stress (in approximately 30% of patients). Other triggers described include a response to eating or to certain head or body positions. The sensation usually improves during periods of relaxation or distraction.

Evaluation and management

All patients should undergo a careful history and physical examination aiming at identifying signs or symptoms of an esophageal motility disorder, especially achalasia. In a recent study of patients with globus sensation, a high proportion of the patients were found to have achalasia. Further diagnostic testing can be performed based upon the severity and duration of symptoms. Endoscopic or barium studies should be obtained in elderly patients, or those with alarm symptoms (such as weight loss, anemia, dysphagia, or odynophagia). Additional work-up may include videofluoroscopic or manometric assessment of esophageal function. Ambulatory pH monitoring may be helpful if reflux is suspected. An empiric trial of acid suppression is a reasonable alternative. Pharmacologic therapy using a tricyclic antidepressant such as imipramine has been beneficial for some patients, particularly those with psychiatric disorders such as panic, somatization, major depression, and agoraphobia.

Prognosis

In a recent study, follow-up of the 88 patients with globus sensation ranging from 3 to 59 months demonstrated that the sensation vanished spontaneously in 13% of those who had received non-specific or no treatment, improved in an additional 25%, and was unchanged in 32%.

Zenker's diverticulum (pharyngoesophageal diverticulum)

Introduction

Zenker and Von Ziemssen first systematically described Zenker's diverticulum, also called pharyngoesophageal diverticulum, in 1877. The precise origin of the diverticulum (between the cricopharynx and the inferior pharyngeal constrictor muscles) was finally identified by Killian at the beginning of the 20th century. Zenker's diverticulum is located above the UES and therefore should be considered as a hypopharyngeal diverticulum. Currently, there is still much controversy regarding the precise cause, pathophysiology, and therapy of Zenker's diverticulum.

Epidemiology

The prevalence of Zenker's diverticulum has been reported to range between 0.01% and 0.11%. The prevalence is higher in the elderly, predominantly in women, with an approximate 50% occurrence in the seventh and eighth decades of life. Zenker's diverticulum is rarely seen in patients younger than 40 years. Zenker's diverticulum grows slowly but continuously.

Etiology

Gastroesophageal reflux disease has been implicated in the genesis of this disorder; this implication is supported by the fact that Zenker's diverticulum is very uncommon in eastern countries where GERD is similarly rare. It has been postulated that acid exposure leads to cricopharyngeal spasm, which will stimulate the development of a pharyngoesophageal diverticulum. Reflux esophagitis, however, as an indicator of GERD, has been reported as rarely associated with Zenker's diverticulum. The association of GERD or UES spasm in the development of the diverticulum is unclear.

More recent studies suggested that the primary pathology responsible for the development of pharyngoesophageal diverticula is the incoordination of cricopharyngeal function. Conversely, others urged that, instead of premature relaxation and contraction of the UES, the pouch is the result of incomplete opening of the UES. Nevertheless, some workers thought these conflicting manometric findings may have been the result of difficulty in properly placing the recording catheter in patients with upper esophageal diverticula.

In a recent report, based on the premise that the poor compliance of the UES in patients with Zenker's diverticulum is the result of muscular, structural changes, muscle strips from Zenker's diverticula were studied histologically and compared with control tissue obtained from autopsy samples of non-dysphagic individuals. The specimens of Zenker's patients showed marked differences, which included fibro-adipose tissue replacement and fiber degeneration. The authors concluded that these fibrous changes might be responsible for the dysphagia and the decreased opening of the UES characteristic of patients with Zenker's diverticulum.

Clinical features

Clinically, Zenker's diverticulum presents, in order of frequency, with

- upper esophageal dysphagia (present in 98% of the cases in one study)
- regurgitation of undigested food
- aspiration
- noisy deglution
- halitosis
- changes in the voice
- mild weight loss may occur.

The most potentially dangerous complications are aspiration and pneumonia (which occur in about 30% of the patients) and perforation. Carcinoma is an unlikely complication (0.48%); when present, however, the long-term survival is nil. Rare cases of massive bleeding in Zenker's diverticula and tracheo-diverticular fistula have been reported. It is common to find associated gastrointestinal pathology that consists of hiatal hernia, gastroduodenal ulcer, midesophageal diverticulum, esophageal spasm, and achalasia.

Diagnosis

Definitive diagnosis of Zenker's diverticulum can be accomplished by a barium esophagram with special attention to the oropharyngeal phase of the swallowing. Endoscopic studies are rarely indicated (and in fact contraindi-cated because of the risk of perforation) although this approach could be useful when carcinoma is suspected on the basis of radiological examinations. In patients with symptomatic disease, the pouches usually have a diameter of more than 2 cm, are typically located in the posterior midline, and generally protrude to the left cervical region (about 10% protrude to the right side). Esophageal manometry is recommended mainly for those patients suspected of additional esophageal motility disorders such as GERD or achalasia.

Treatment

Small Zenker's diverticula discovered by chance may be followed by periodic esophagrams. Patients suffering from transient diverticula are usually asymptomatic and require no treatment. These diverticula should be regarded as incidental findings in patients without upper esophageal symptoms. The solution for larger pharyngoesophageal diverticulum is surgical. Today, in contrast with earlier views, there is consensus that every large diverticulum should be surgically managed, given its certain progression in size, symptomatology, and potential for complications.

A diversity of surgical techniques has been proposed for the correction of this disorder. Very early reports proposed a two-stage operation in which the neck of the diverticulum was ligated, and the pouch was attached to the skin and irrigated until eventual spontaneous closure occurred. A later modification consisted of suturing the diverticulum to the skin and removing the pouch 2 weeks later. This modification afforded lower morbidity and mortality. In addition, one-stage resection of pharyngoesophageal diverticula became widely accepted until the late 1960s. Cricopharyngeal myotomy was then introduced as a technique based on previous reports on myotomy with or without resection of the pouch. Excellent results have been reported in different studies with the use of myotomy alone, obviating the need for sutures and eliminating leakage risk.

Currently, it is generally agreed that better results are obtained by diverticulopexy combined with extramucosal myotomy of the UES. After diverticulopexy, oral feedings can be resumed immediately. However, it is worth delaying feeding for a few days if diverticulectomy was performed. It is possible for salivary fistulas to ensue, in which case oral feedings should be withheld and total parenteral nutrition initiated. Fistulas usually heal in about 2 weeks, after which oral feedings can be resumed.

An innovative modification of this technique includes endoscopic stapling of the diverticulum. This technique uses an endosurgical stapler that simultaneously divides the wall between the esophagus and the pouch and staples the wound edges closed. The advantages of this approach include optimal hemostasis, no cervical space contamination, and avoidance of perforation at the bottom of the diverticulum, besides being relatively cheaper than the laser approach. Further trials with larger series are necessary before endoscopic stapling is definitely adopted as the treatment of choice for Zenker's diverticulum.

Primary esophageal motility disorders

Achalasia

Achalasia is a long-recognized primary esophageal motility disorder characterized by a distinct set of manometric and radiographic findings. The primary motility problems in achalasia are a failure of the LES to relax completely during swallowing and a failure of the esophageal smooth muscle to generate effective peristalsis.

Pathogenesis

The definitive cause of achalasia is unknown, but smooth muscle denervation is thought to be responsible for the motility abnormalities. This hypothesis is consistent with the observation that patients suffering from Chagas' disease have strikingly similar esophageal motility abnormalities as those with achalasia. However, pathologic findings in achalasia are also present in the central nervous system such as the dorsal motor nucleus of the vagus. Eight neuropathologic findings have been described in achalasia:

1. in early achalasia inflammation of the myenteric plexus without a decrease in ganglionic cells or neurofibrosis
2. in a later stage loss of ganglionic cells starts
3. a decrease in varicose nerve fibers of the myenteric plexus
4. degenerative changes of the vagus nerve
5. quantitative and qualitative changes in the dorsal motor nucleus of the vagus nerve
6. marked decreases in small intramuscular nerve fibers, as well as a decrease in vasointestinal peptide (VIP) and neuropeptide Y immunostaining of the nerve fibers
7. paucity of vesicles in small nerve fibers
8. occasional presence of intracytoplasmic inclusions (Lewy bodies) in the dorsal motor nucleus of the vagus and myenteric plexus.

About 1% of achalasia cases are familial. Most of these cases are horizontally transmitted, occurring in the pediatric group and between siblings and twins. The likely mode of inheritance in these cases is autosomal recessive, with full penetrance in the homozygotic form. A small proportion of the familial achalasia cases are vertically transmitted. This form of familial achalasia appears to affect older patients.

Another 1% of achalasia cases appear to be associated with degenerative neurologic diseases such as Parkinson's disease and hereditary cerebellar ataxia. One study noted Lewy bodies in degenerating ganglionic cells of the myenteric plexus and vagal dorsal motor nucleus in patients with achalasia and Parkinson's disease. Other case reports also linked achalasia with hereditary cerebellar ataxia.

The remaining 98% of the achalasia cases are so-called "idiopathic achalasia". There are two main postulated etiologies to idiopathic achalasia based on limited and indirect evidence; these are autoimmune and infectious. Several studies suggested an autoimmune etiology. Achalasia has been found to be associated with a class II histocompatibility antigen, Dqw1, which is implicated in autoimmune processes. In addition, monocytic infiltration of myenteric ganglionic cells and myenteric inflammation occur in patients with early achalasia. Furthermore, 39% to 64% of achalasia patients have serum antibodies against neurons of the myenteric plexus, while less than 8% of normal subjects possess these autoantibodies. With regard to the infectious etiology, several studies have reported a higher measles or varicellar-zoster titer in patients with achalasia compared to controls. Overall, the evidence supporting the autoimmune and infectious hypotheses has been very limited and circumstantial.

Clinical features

Achalasia can present at any age from birth to the ninth decade of life. It is relatively rare during the first two decades of life. Mean age for achalasia in case series ranged between 30 and 60 years, with a peak in the fourth decade. The incidence of achalasia is 0.4 to 1.1 per 100 000 and the prevalence is about 7.9 to 12.6 per 100 000. Patients with achalasia often present with symptoms of chest pain, regurgitation, and dysphagia. Unlike other esophageal motility disorders such as diffuse esophageal spasm (DES) and nutcracker esophagus, which also cause chest pain or dysphagia, achalasia may become progressively severe and may be associated with weight loss.

Dysphagia is the most common and prominent symptom. Solid-food dysphagia is accompanied by varying degrees of liquid dysphagia, although the onset of dysphagia is usually confined at first to solids but later involves liquids. In many patients, the dysphagia seemed to increase in severity over time. In a small number of patients, dysphagia could remain mild for years without significant progression. The degree of dysphagia can be assessed by asking the patient to compare the lengths of time it takes to eat a similar meal before and after the onset of dysphagia. Patients also employ adaptive behaviors to ameliorate the symptom. Classic ones include

1. head-back position while maintaining an upright posture associated with a Valsalva maneuver
2. drinking carbonated beverages
3. belching
4. drinking alcoholic or warm liquids.

Substernal chest pain is noted in 42% of patients with achalasia. The pain is described as a squeezing, pressure-like sensation substernally, at times radiating to the neck, arm, jaws, and back, occurring postprandially or nocturnally. Chest pain tends to be seen more frequently in younger achalasia patients, and is less likely to be associated with dysphagia, regurgitation, and weight loss. Classic pyrosis (heartburn) is noted in 42% of patients with achalasia. This symptom is generally not relieved by antacids, usually does not occur postprandially, and is not associated with abnormal 24-hour pH studies. Therefore, in patients with heartburn refractory to acid-suppression therapy, achalasia should be excluded.

Achalasia patients may also have other symptoms related to retention of solids or liquids in the esophagus when severe impairment of esophageal clearance is present. For example, patients may report regurgitation of undigested food or awakening with undigested food on the pillow. The regurgitated food is described as non-bilious and generally non-acidic. Patients usually adapt to this problem by elevating the head of the bed at night and refrain from eating large meals prior to bedtime. Episodes of aspiration pneumonia may occur for similar reasons.

Weight loss is noted in 84% of patients but with marked variability. In general, weight loss is a marker of severe achalasia. Weight gain after treatment, on the other hand, is a good gauge of improved esophageal clearance.

Complications of achalasia occur in a small proportion of patients. Most of these patients have long-standing disease and dilated esophagi. Three major physiologic processes underlie these complications.

1. displacement of mediastinal structure by the esophagus
2. esophageal ulceration or perforation
3. aspiration of esophageal content.

Furthermore, patients with achalasia are sixteen times more likely to develop esophageal cancer than people without achalasia.

Diagnosis

The classic manometric findings in achalasia are a lack of primary peristalsis and incomplete LES relaxation in response to a wet swallow. Another associated finding is hypertensive LES (normal resting LES pressure does not rule out achalasia). A subset of patients may have simultaneous high-amplitude repetitive contractions on manometry; they are classified as having vigorous achalasia. Early or "incomplete" achalasia may present with hypertensive LES syndrome, incomplete LES relaxation or poor peristalsis alone. In these cases, the diagnosis of achalasia cannot be made on the basis of manometric findings alone.

Barium swallow is immensely helpful in confirming the diagnosis of achalasia and providing information with regard to its severity (Figure 4.1). Classic findings include a dilated esophagus with a fluid level and a tapering of the distal esophagus to a "bird's-beak" configuration. The distal narrowing reflects an LES

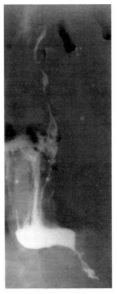

Figure 4.1 Achalasia. Note the markedly dilated esophagus with food debris and air admixed with barium. The distal esophagus has a tapered appearance (Bird's Beak), leading to the lower esophageal sphincter that is unable to relax.

that is unable to relax. In the dilated esophagus, retained food could be seen admixed with barium. Aperistalsis can be demonstrated by fluoroscopy.

Upper endoscopy usually confirms the presence of retained food in a dilated esophagus with a tight LES. Advancing the endoscope with gentle and steady pressure, endoscopists can usually overcome the LES pressure and "pop through" the narrowing. Upper endoscopy is useful in ruling out lesions such as malignancies. Patients who appear to have evidence of external esophageal compression should be further evaluated by endoscopic ultrasound or chest computed tomography (CT) or magnetic resonance imaging (MRI).

Management of achalasia

Management of achalasia consists of three modalities: botulinum toxin injection, balloon dilation, and surgery. Oral medications have a minimal role in the treatment of achalasia, as calcium channel blockers and nitrates aimed at reducing LES pressure are generally either ineffective or have short-lived effectiveness.

Endoscopic botulinum toxin injection into the LES has been shown to improve LES relaxation and decrease esophageal transit time significantly in patients with achalasia. The mean duration of symptomatic response to bolulinum toxin injection is about 4 months with marked variations from one patient to another. The response may be longer in elderly patients. Therefore, this may be a preferred modality in this population who may have high surgical risks or in whom a relatively easy but temporary solution is desired.

Esophageal dilation has been used to treat achalasia for hundreds of years. Currently it is performed during upper endoscopy with fluoroscopic guidance. Only pneumatic balloon dilators can be used. About 40% of patients report improvement after one session of dilation, lasting 5 years. Duration of response is highly variable. Many patients need periodic dilation on an as-needed basis. Esophageal dilation is associated with a 5% risk of perforation and bleeding.

Surgical treatment of achalasia involves an LES myotomy. This procedure has been modified over the past few decades. It basically involves one or more incisions made at the gastroesophageal junction to sever the muscle fiber and thereby relieve the LES pressure. Laparoscopic LES myotomy has been developed recently. Furthermore, in an effort to prevent gastroesophageal reflux following LES myotomy, anti-reflux fundoplication procedures are usually performed concurrently with the myotomy. In a long-term randomized trial, most (95%) patients undergoing surgical myotomy were almost symptom free at 5 years, as compared to only 51% of those who received dilation. Myotomy is associated with complications such as strictures. Incomplete myotomy may lead to recurrent dysphagia.

Secondary achalasia

It is important to consider the possibility of other esophageal conditions that could produce a similar radiographical appearance as achalasia (Box 4.2). For example, neoplasms of the esophagus, stomach and mediastinum can cause so-called pseudo-achalasia, mimicking primary achalasia. They may occur through one of two mechanisms: direct LES obstruction by the tumor or as a paraneoplastic antibody-mediated disorder. Other diseases that are associated with achalasia-like motility disorders are listed in Table 4.1.

Diffuse esophageal spasm

Diffuse esophageal spasm is a relatively rare diagnosis among patients undergoing esophageal manometry for dysphagia or chest pain, accounting for only about 3% of these patients. DES can be seen at any age, although most commonly patients are over the age of 50 years. Its prevalence is equal in the both sexes.

Pathophysiology

The pathophysiology of DES is unknown. Several studies have shown that the esophagus of patients with DES is hypersensitive to cholinergic and hormonal stimulation. In addition, recent data have suggested that the low

Box 4.2 Diseases mimicking achalasia
Neoplasms of the esophagus, stomach, and mediastinum

Amyloidosis
Sarcoidosis
Chagas' disease
Eosinophilic gastroenteritis
Neurofibromatosis
Idiopathic intestinal pseudo-obstruction
Anderson–Fabry's disease
Multiple endocrine neoplasia, type IIB

levels of nitric oxide, a neurotransmitter, may be responsible for the uncoordinated contractions in DES. Furthermore, familial clustering has been reported, suggesting a possible genetic link for this disorder in some individuals. Others have suggested that DES is closely related to achalasia. Indeed several documented cases of DES have evolved into achalasia.

Clinical features

Clinically, patients usually present with chest pain and dysphagia. The chest pain can vary from mild to severe, lasting from seconds to minutes, and often radiating to the back. The pain does not always occur with swallowing. The chest pain can often be relieved by nitroglycerin, mimicking cardiac angina, however, the pain is rarely exertional. The dysphagia can be associated with solids or liquids, and can often be induced by stress, rapid eating, and cold or other irritating foods. In contrast to the dysphagia in achalasia, the dysphagia in DES is intermittent and non-progressive. Aspiration or regurgitation is usually not seen with DES. Food impaction and fear of eating have been reported in patients with DES.

Diagnosis

The diagnosis of DES requires radiographical and manometric studies. The classic barium swallow findings of DES are the "corkscrew" appearance of the esophageal body (Figure 4.2), reflecting a simultaneous contraction and severe tertiary activity. Normal peristalsis is usually seen in the upper third of the esophagus. Abnormal primary peristalsis is often seen distal to the aortic arch. The LES region is usually normal manometrically. Interestingly, episodes of pain do not always correlate with esophageal spasm, raising the question whether the manometric and radiographic evidence of contractions are the real underlying abnormalities responsible for the symptoms. In addition, many examinations are normal.

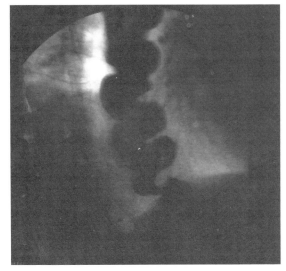

Figure 4.2 "Corkscrew" esophagus in a patient with diffuse esophageal spasm.

Esophageal manometry is the only way to accurately make the diagnosis of DES. Manometrically, DES is defined as simultaneous contractions in 20% or greater of wet swallows intermixed with normal peristalsis in the distal esophagus with contraction amplitude exceeding 30 mmHg. It is important to recognize that simultaneous contractions may be seen in other diseases such as diabetes mellitus, scleroderma, amyloidosis, idiopathic pseudo-obstruction, alcoholic neuropathies, and GERD. The findings of prolonged or multi-peaked contractions support the diagnosis of DES. High-amplitude DES is more likely to be seen in patients with chest pain, while low-amplitude DES is more often observed in patients with dysphagia.

Prognosis

In long-term follow-up studies, the prognosis of patients with DES is excellent. Transition to classic achalasia has been reported to be 3% to 5% of cases, while some investigators believe that true DES is part of the continuum of achalasia. Symptoms generally remain stable or resolve spontaneously over time. Diffuse esophageal spasm has not been associated with the development of malignancies.

Hypercontractile esophagus (nutcracker esophagus and hypertensive lower esophageal sphincter)

High-amplitude contractions in the esophageal body (in excess of 180 mmHg) are named "nutcracker esophagus". Another type of hypercontractile esophageal abnormality is hypertensive LES. Hypertensive LES is defined manometrically as a resting pressure greater than 45 mmHg. These two hypercontractile abnormalities often occur simultaneously, suggesting that they may share a common etiology.

Nutcracker esophagus is seen predominantly in patients with non-cardiac chest pain. Between 27% to 48% of patients evaluated for non-cardiac chest pain meet the diagnostic criteria for nutcracker esophagus. Hypertensive LES is a relatively uncommon manometric abnormality that is also typically seen in patients being evaluated for chest pain and dysphagia. These manometric findings are often non-specific and should not be issued as specific diagnoses as they have both been reported in patients with GERD. In addition, a causal relationship between these manometric findings and symptoms such as chest pain is poorly established.

Pathophysiology

The etiology of nutcracker esophagus or hypertensive LES is unknown. Nutcracker esophagus is analogous in many respects to irritable bowel syndrome in that patients with nutcracker esophagus share a similar psychiatric profile with patients with irritable bowel syndrome. Specifically, patients with nutcracker

esophagus have a decreased pain threshold for esophageal balloon distension compared with normal subjects. This is similar to the low pain threshold to rectal distension in irritable bowel syndrome patients. Finally, patients with nutcracker esophagus also are more likely to suffer from other functional bowel symptoms. Psychological abnormalities have also been described in patients with hypertensive LES, suggesting a stress-related component and overlap with nutcracker esophagus. It is possible that nutcracker esophagus and hypertensive LES represent two entities along the same spectrum of hypercontractile dysmotility of the distal esophagus. A significant proportion of patients with hypertensive LES or nutcracker esophagus are shown to have abnormal esophageal reflux by 24-hour pH studies. However, it is not clear whether these two entities are linked to GERD. Rarely, patients with nutcracker esophagus can progress to develop achalasia.

Clinical features

Ninety per cent of patients with nutcracker esophagus present with chest pain. The intensity, location, and frequency of the symptom vary. Most patients with nutcracker esophagus are referred by an internist or a cardiologist after negative cardiac work-up for chest pain. Depression, anxiety disorder, and somatization are commonly associated symptoms. Dysphagia is uncommon in nutcracker esophagus, but may be seen with hypertensive LES.

Diagnosis

Barium study of the esophagus in patients with nutcracker esophagus or hypertensive LES is generally normal, although tertiary waves are occasionally present. The diagnosis of nutcracker esophagus relies on esophageal manometry. The manometric criteria of nutcracker esophagus require that the contraction amplitude must be greater than 180 mmHg in over 90% of the contractions and that all contractions must be peristaltic. The location of the manometric abnormality is generally seen in the smooth-muscle portion of the esophagus. However, it can involve only the distal esophagus.

Prognosis

The clinical importance of nutcracker esoph-agus and hypertensive LES is a matter of con-troversy at this point. As a result, reassurance can provide significant relief of symptoms in many patients.

Treatment of diffuse esophageal spasm and hypercontractile motility disorders

Diffuse esophageal spasm, hypertensive LES, and nutcracker esophagus are usually non-progressive disorders that have good prognosis. Once cardiac disease has been excluded, the treatment should aim to relieve symptoms. Patient education, reassurance, and establish-ment of a good patient–doctor rapport can often lead to significant improvement in symptoms. Many patients may experience spontaneous improvement or resolution of symptoms in the absence of treatment.

Pharmacology Trazodone, an anxiolytic medication, is the only agent that has been shown to improve symptoms of spastic disor-ders of the esophagus in a prospective, blind-ed, controlled trial. Muscle relaxants such as nitrates, calcium channel blockers, and even botulinum toxin have been used to treat DES and nutcracker esophagus. However, the reported clinical response is limited to case reports and case series. Some investiga-tors have also advocated treating these patients with anti–reflux agents based on the observation that the frequency of abnormal esophageal pH is high among patients with nutcracker esophagus. More recently, low-dose tricyclic antidepressants have been used.

Endoscopy Studies evaluating esophageal dilation in patients with DES and nutcracker esophagus are limited by a placebo effect. There are limited data on botulinum toxin for DES and nutcracker esophagus. Neither treatment can be generally recommended at this point unless there are achalasia-like features.

Surgery The available data on surgical myotomy in DES and nutcracker esophagus suggest a trend toward symptomatic relief in the subgroup of patients with severe refracto-ry symptoms. However, none of the studies was a controlled trial. Surgical myotomy should not be considered in patients with refractory and severe symptoms in light of the unproven benefit and the potential for adverse effects.

Hypocontractile esophagus

A more commonly used term for this catego-ry of esophageal motility disorders is "ineffec-tive esophageal motility". A number of manometrically different findings are collec-tively described as ineffective esophageal motility: low-amplitude (<30 mmHg) peri-staltic contractions, non-transmission of the peristaltic sequence (drop-out of the sequence), or low-amplitude simultaneous contraction in the distal esophagus. These dif-ferent types of motility abnormalities all lead to ineffective transport of food boluses through the esophagus. It has been speculated that long-term distal esophageal acid expo-sure in chronic GERD patients may be responsible for the increased prevalence of ineffective esophageal motility and hypoten-sive LES observed in this patient population. Although several studies demonstrated a strong link between ineffective esophageal motility and GERD, a more recent retrospec-tive study failed to demonstrate such an association.

Secondary esophageal motility abnormalities

The esophageal motility disorders in this category are due to either esophageal injuries or a systemic disease. The prototypic secondary esophageal motility disorder is seen in patients with scleroderma. Abnormal connective tissue infiltration leads to abnormal smooth muscle function. Chagas' disease due to *Trypanosoma cruzi* produces an achalasia-like motility disorder. Autonomic neuropathy associated with diabetes mellitus gives rise to distinctly abnormal esophageal motility, sometimes resembling diffuse esophageal spasm. Loss of peristalsis in the distal esophagus can often be seen in chronic idiopathic intestinal pseudo-obstruction, amyloidosis and hypothyroidism. A detailed discussion of esophageal involvement of scleroderma is given below.

Scleroderma

Scleroderma is a systemic connective tissue disease characterized by obliterative small-vessel vasculitis and proliferation of connective tissue. Scleroderma can involve the skin, kidney, heart, lungs, and gastrointestinal tract. Gastrointestinal-tract involvement occurs in up to 90% of patients with scleroderma. The esophagus is the most frequently affected gastrointestinal tract segment in scleroderma.

Pathology The pathologic changes seen in the esophagus with advanced scleroderma involvement include smooth muscle atrophy, sclerosis of arterioles, and collagen deposition in the lamina propria, submucosa, and serosa. These advanced pathologic changes are probably preceded by esophageal neuronal abnormalities that are characterized by a clinically latent period of cholinergic neural dysfunction. Recent studies employing endoscopic ultrasonography also suggested that fibrosis in the muscularis propria of scleroderma esophagus may be prominent and play a major part in causing the functional esophageal abnormalities in scleroderma.

Clinical features Esophageal manifestations in patients with scleroderma mainly consist of pyrosis, regurgitation, and dysphagia. Gastroesophageal reflux disease is responsible for the pyrosis experienced by patients with scleroderma. Patients with scleroderma esophagus are prone to gastroesophageal reflux for two reasons: poor or absent distal esophageal peristalsis, and low LES pressure. The degree of distal esophageal acid exposure is determined by both the severity of distal esophageal aperistalsis and the degree of LES hypotension. While GERD is common in patients with scleroderma esophagus, the available data suggest that there may be increased incidence of GERD-related complications such as peptic stricture, Barrett's esophagus, and esophageal adenocarcinoma in this patient population. The dysphagia associated with scleroderma esophagus can be due to many reasons including esophageal dysmotility, benign GERD-related peptic stricture, erosive esophagitis, and esophageal adenocarcinoma.

Diagnosis The diagnosis of scleroderma is based on clinical criteria established by the American Rheumatism Association. Evidence of esophageal involvement can be confirmed by radiographical and manometric studies. Lateral chest radiograph may show an air esophagram and a dilated and atonic esophagus visualized as a prominent air-filled structure. Air esophagram is not specific for scleroderma, but is more commonly seen in patients with achalasia. When it occurs in patients with scleroderma esophagus, the possibility of a distal esophageal obstruction should be excluded. Barium esophagram usually reveals esophageal dilation and a patulous gastroesophageal junction with evidence of free reflux. The primary peristalsis is often absent or diminished in the smooth-muscle portion of the esophagus. Evidence of erosive

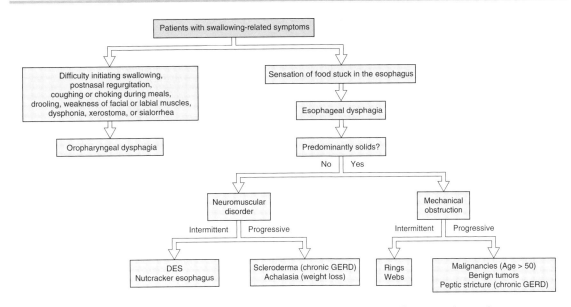

Figure 4.3 Diagnostic approach for patients with dysphagia. DES diffuse esophageal spasm (adapted from Castell DO, Richter JE, eds. *The Esophagus* 3rd edn, Philadelphia: Lippincott Williams and Wilkins; 2000).

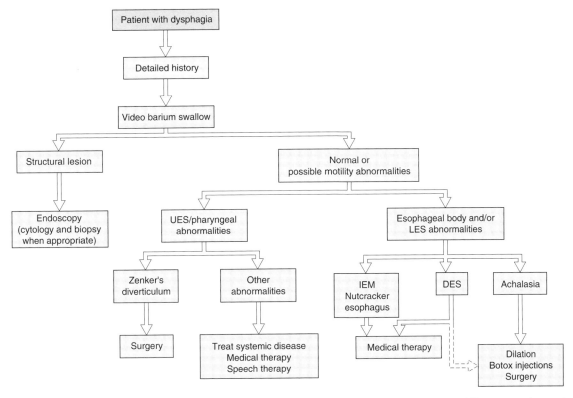

Figure 4.4 Diagnostic work-up for patients presenting with dysphagia. DES diffuse esophageal spasm, IEM ineffective esophageal motility (adapted from Castell DO, Richter JE, eds. *The Esophagus* 3rd edn, Philadelphia: Lippincott Williams and Wilkins; 2000).

esophagitis and distal esophageal stricture may be identified.

Manometric findings Up to 90% of patients with scleroderma have esophageal manometric abnormalities. Typical manometric findings include decreased frequency or amplitude of peristalsis, or aperistalsis in the distal smooth-muscle portion of the esophagus, and preserved peristalsis in the proximal striated muscle portion. Early scleroderma may not show these findings or only mild abnormalities. Hypotensive LES is a common finding. The combination of compromised distal esophageal peristalsis and hypotensive LES on manometry can also be seen in other diseases including hypothyroidism, myositis, intestinal pseudo-obstruction, and severe long-standing GERD.

Management of esophageal involvement of scleroderma There is no disease-modifying agent for scleroderma that has been shown to clearly improve esophageal peristalsis or LES dysfunction. Therefore, the focus of the management of esophageal dysfunction in patients with scleroderma centers on suppression of acid and enhancing gastric emptying. With the advent of potent acid-suppression medications such as the proton pump inhibitors, control of GERD can be achieved in the vast majority of patients. Anti-reflux surgery should be considered with great caution in the few patients who fail medical anti-reflux treatment because of the high risk of worsening dysphagia and further delay in gastric emptying.

Further reading

Adler DG, Romero Y. Primary esophageal motility disorders. *Mayo Clin Proc* 2001; 76: 195–200.

Castell DO, Richter JE, eds. *The Esophagus* 3rd edn, Philadelphia, PA: Lippincott Williams & Wilkins; 2000.

Cook IJ, Kahrilas PJ. AGA technical review on management of oropharyngeal dysphagia. *Gastroenterology* 1999; 116: 455–478.

Hirano I, Tatum RP, Shi G, *et al*. Manometric heterogeneity in patients with idiopathic achalasia. *Gastroenterology* 2001; 120: 789.

Kahrilas PJ. Esophageal motility disorders: current concepts of pathogenesis and treatment. *Can J Gastroenterol* 2000; 14: 221–231.

Lock G, Holstege A, Lang B, *et al*. Gastrointestinal manifestations of progressive systemic sclerosis. *Am J Gastroenterol* 1997; 92: 763–771.

Rothstein R. A systematic approach to a patient with dysphagia. *Hosp Pract* 1997; 32: 169.

Spechler SJ and Castell DO. Classification of esophageal motility abnormalities. *Gut* 2001; 49: 145–151.

Spechler SJ. AGA technical review on treatment of patients with dysphagia caused by benign disorders of the distal esophagus. *Gastroenterology* 1999; 117: 233–254.

Trate DM, Parkman HP, Fisher RS. Dysphagia: evaluation, diagnosis and treatment. *Prim Care* 1996; 23: 417.

Chapter 5

Transfer Dysphagia

Natasha Mirza, Cesar Ruiz and Patricia Dooley

CHAPTER OUTLINE

Definition

Disturbances affecting the biomechanics of swallowing secondary to any pathology proximal to the esophagus are known as transfer dysphagia. This condition is also known as oropharyngeal dysphagia, and has a high morbidity, mortality, and cost. It is very common in the chronic-care setting and is seen in more than half of all patients who reside in nursing homes. Detailed examination of the anatomy and physiology of each stage of deglutition is necessary to effectively diagnose and treat this form of dysphagia.

Anatomy and physiology of the swallowing mechanism

Normal swallowing is a complex mechanism involving many levels of the central nervous system and voluntary and involuntary muscles in the head and neck. There are three phases of swallowing, each involving a particular subset of anatomic structures and muscle activity, they are the

1. oral phase
2. pharyngeal phase
3. esophageal phase.

We will now discuss the anatomy of the structures involved in each phase (see Figure 5.1).

The structures involved in the oropharyngeal aspect of swallowing are as follows (see Figure 5.2):

- lips
- dentition

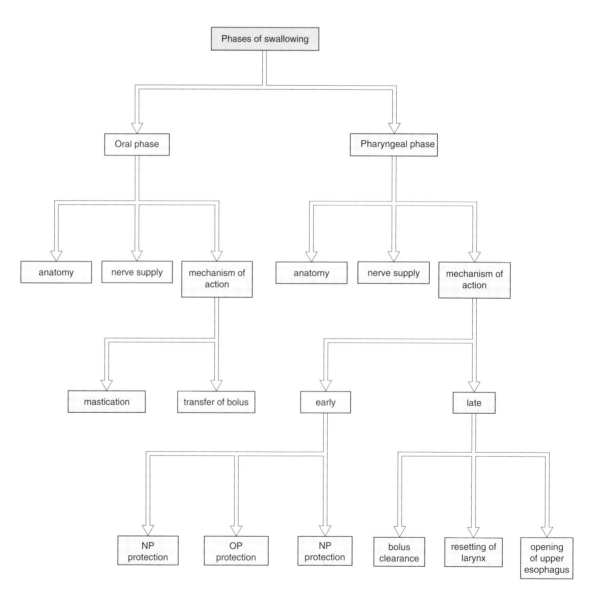

Figure 5.1 Phases of swallowing.

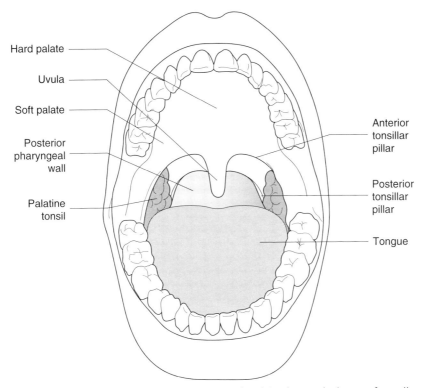

Figure 5.2 View of the oral cavity and structures involved in the oral phase of swallowing.

- tongue
- palate
- salivary glands
- pharyngeal muscles.

Lips

The mimetic muscles involved are the orbicularis oris, levator labii superioris, depressor labii inferioris, and the mentalis. The sensory nerve supply of the lips is from branches of the maxillary division of the trigeminal nerve and the motor supply to these muscles, as well as to the rest of the face, is via the facial nerve.

Dentition and structures involved in mastication

The maxillary and mandibular teeth are responsible for biting and mastication. The muscles that help with chewing are the masseterics, temporalis, medial pterygoids, and lateral pterygoids. They are all supplied by the mandibular branch of the trigeminal nerve. The other masticatory muscles are the suprahyoid group of muscles including the mylohyoid, stylohyoid, geniohyoid and digastric muscles. The pterygoid plates and the sphenoid bones act as anchors for the masseteric muscles to act on. The suprahyoid muscle group elevates the larynx and help further in swallowing.

Tongue

The intrinsic muscles of the tongue are the longtitudinal, transverse, vertical, and oblique muscles. They are primarily responsible for producing the changes in the shape of the tongue during swallowing. The extrinsic muscles are the genioglossus, hyoglossus, palatoglossus, and styloglossus. These muscles are responsible for pulling the tongue forward, backward, upward, and downward. The nerve supply to all the lingual muscles is from the hypoglossal cranial nerve except for the palatoglossus which is supplied by a branch of the vagus.

Palate

The anterior hard palate is the palatine bone and palatine process of the maxilla covered by mucosa. The posterior soft palate is a fibromuscular shelf with salivary glands. The muscles include the tensor veli palatini and its aponeurosis, the palatopharyngeus, levator veli palatini, musculus uvulae, and the palatoglossus. The sensory nerve to the palate is the vidian nerve arising from the maxillary division of the

trigeminal, and the motor nerves are from the pharyngeal plexus composed of glossopharyngeal and vagal branches (Figure 5.3).

Salivary glands

The major glands are the parotid glands, and the submandibular and sublingual glands. Besides these there are several hundred minor salivary glands scattered all over the oral cavity. The minor glands produce a basal salivary secretion for lubrication and dental hygiene. The major glands are reflexogenic in nature and produce large amounts of mucoid or serous saliva in response to food or irritation.

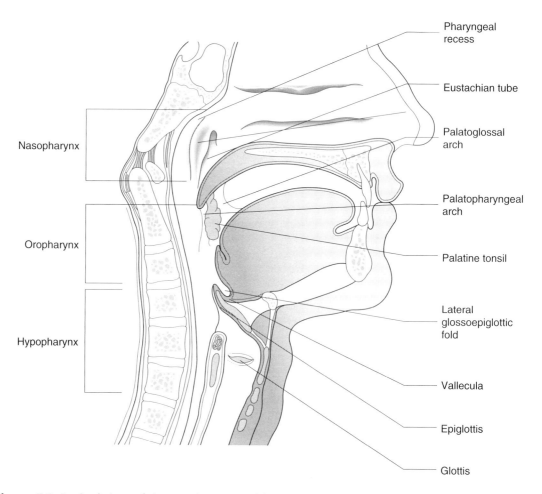

Figure 5.3 Sagittal view of the oropharynx and larynx and structures involved in the oral and pharyngeal phases of swallowing.

The nerve supply to the major glands is via parasympathetic nerves including branches of the glossopharyngeal and facial nerves. The superior and inferior salivatory nuclei in the midbrain are the centers for this parasympathetic supply.

Taste

The sensory nerves involved in taste are the chorda tympani branch of the facial nerve over the anterior two-thirds of the tongue and the glossopharyngeal nerve posteriorly. Most posteriorly some branches of the vagus nerve also carry taste fibers.

Pharyngeal muscles

These comprise structures extending superiorly from the base of the skull to the posterior surface of the base of the cricoid cartilage inferiorly. The pharynx is a funnel-shaped muscular tube lined by mucous membrane and is approximately 12 cm long. Anteriorly it opens into the nasal cavity, the oral cavity below that, and finally in the posterior aspect of the larynx. The superior, middle, and inferior constrictor muscles form the muscular tube. Posteriorly it abuts the pharyngobasilar fascia, prevertebral muscles, and the cervical muscles. The sensory and motor nerve supply to these muscles is from the pharyngeal plexus comprising the glossopharyngeal and vagus nerves and some branches of the facial nerve. The stylohyoid, stylopharyngeus, palatopharyngeus, and salpingopharyngeus muscles suspend the pharynx from the base of the skull. At some sites there are mucosal folds and grooves which further help direct the food bolus in the right direction. These include the glossoepiglottic folds and below these the two recesses along either side of the larynx called the piriform sinuses (see Figures 5.4 and 5.5).

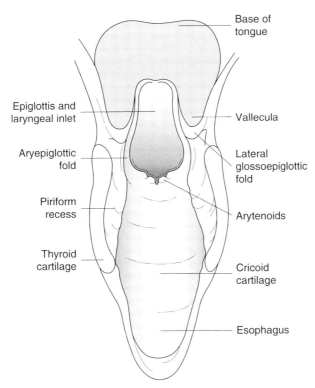

Figure 5.4 Posterior view of the larynx showing the base of tongue and piriform sinuses.

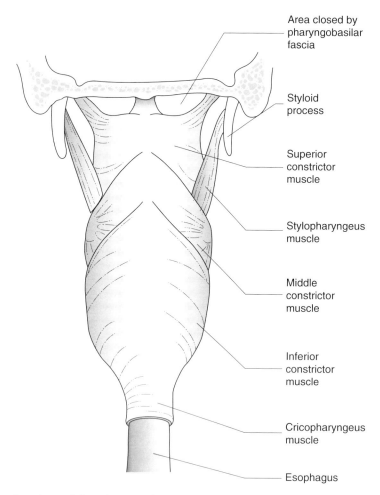

Figure 5.5 Posterior view of the pharynx showing the constrictor muscles.

Mechanism of swallowing

Oral phase

This consists of the oral preparatory stage and the actual oral stage. It involves the intake, mastication, and the transfer of the food bolus from the mouth to the pharynx. See Figure 5.6 for the neurological control of swallowing.

Control of the swallowing mechanism is in the higher centers of the cortex and involves stimulation by the sight, smell, and taste of food. From there impulses are transmitted to the center located in the reticular formation of the brainstem. Impulses arrive at this medullary center via sensory afferent nerves. Most of this sensory input is processed in the nucleus tractus solitarius. Motor efferents then emanate from the nucleus ambiguus. The swallowing cascade once initiated is reflexogenic and cannot be stopped. It may be overridden however by central influences. Respiration is inhibited centrally during the process of swallowing. Subsequent to the initiation of swallowing a complex process of coordination occurs between the tongue, pharynx, and UES.

Oral preparatory stage

This phase involves
- lip closure
- jaw motion
- buccal and facial tone

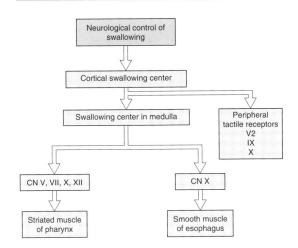

Figure 5.6 Neurological control of swallowing.

- tongue movement
- bulging of the soft palate.

The first step involves the biting of a food morsel by the teeth. The lips are then closed and the front of the mouth is sealed by the tip of the tongue. This requires the lip musculature to come into play and produce retraction, protrusion, and a pursing action.

The teeth and the masticatory muscles then work to grind the food. The jaw movement in a lateral and rotary fashion assists with molar mastication. Similar rotary and lateral motion of the tongue is critical in controlling the bolus in the mouth and placing it on the teeth. Lubrication and some digestive function is provided by the reflex secretion from the salivary glands. The larynx and pharynx are at rest during this phase. The airway is open and nasal breathing may continue until the voluntary swallow is initiated.

Acute oral stage

A bolus of suitable size and consistency is created and then transferred posteriorly from the oral cavity to the pharynx. The tip of the tongue is placed against the maxillary incisors and the tongue forms a trough into which the food is placed. The bolus is thrust backward by the patterned contractions of the lingual muscles. The soft palate is bulged anteriorly and widens the nasal airway and narrows the oropharyngeal inlet thereby decreasing the possibility of premature spillage of food into the pharynx. This is further assisted by salivary lubrication. This salivary secretion is induced by the tactile and taste stimuli provided by food in the mouth. The food is thus broken down to a consistency suitable for swallowing.

Pharyngeal phase

The pharyngeal phase of swallowing is involuntary and under reflex control. The bolus, along with contact of the tongue with the faucial pillars, stimulates receptors in the oropharynx which trigger the pharyngeal swallow. Also the pressure force of the bolus is responsible for the initiation of this stage. In order for this phase to begin it is necessary to have something in the mouth, either food, liquid, or saliva. Normally during this transit through the pharynx the bolus does not hesitate and a smooth movement is observed. It consists of two periods – the early protective period and the later period which lasts less than 1 second.

Early period

Nasopharyngeal protection In this phase the bolus is thrust posteriorly by the tongue. The pharynx is elevated and develops a fold called the "ridge of Passavant". The soft palate also elevates and meets the ridge thereby sealing off the nasopharynx. The three pharyngeal constrictors then contract from above downward thus stripping remains of the bolus into the relaxed lower portion of the pharynx and hence into the esophagus.

Oropharyngeal protection The peristaltic action of the constrictors is such that the bolus is propelled downward and is not allowed to regurgitate back into the oral cavity.

Laryngeal protection There are three parts to this very vital protective function.

1. Laryngeal elevation occurs from the contraction of the suprahyoid musculature and the larynx moves up and under the base of the tongue.
2. Following this the epiglottis folds backward and downward and the valleculae at the back of the tongue are emptied of food. The bolus is diverted around the piriform recesses. The epiglottis, however, does not fit tightly enough over the larynx to entirely prevent the entrance of liquids and food.
3. At this point the laryngeal sphincters come into play. There is adduction of the true vocal cords followed by adduction of the false cords and the aryepiglottic folds. This closure of the vocal cords is the most critical event in the prevention of aspiration. The bolus is thereby diverted into the lateral piriform recesses.

Later period

At rest the cricoid lamina touches the posterior pharyngeal wall at the level of the cricopharyngeal region. This position of the cricoid maintains closure of the UES. As the larynx elevates and moves anteriorly during the swallow, extrinsic stretch is placed on the cricopharyngeus muscle and its adjacent fibers. The muscular components of the valve contribute to the opening and separation of the cricoid lamina from the posterior pharyngeal wall and account for the opening of the cricopharyngeal region. The bolus is now cleared by the stripping action of the superior, middle and inferior constrictor muscles. There is resetting of the larynx and the upper esophagus now opens by the relaxation of the cricopharyngeus muscle. This muscle normally stays closed between swallows and during inspiration. Momentary relaxation occurs immediately in advance of the descending bolus and only fully relaxes when there is full glottic closure.

When the bolus is cleared there is a resetting of the swallowing mechanism which involves relaxation of the soft palate, tongue, and pharynx. The larynx returns to its resting position and the epiglottis snaps back into its upright position.

Esophageal phase

This phase involves active peristalsis or sequential contraction from top to bottom in two waves, primary peristalsis and secondary peristalsis. The esophageal phase is under involuntary neural control. At the base of the esophagus the LES is a circular muscular valve that opens to allow the passage of food but is otherwise closed to prevent gastroesophageal reflux. Structurally and physiologically the LES is different from the UES. The esophageal phase is not amenable to any therapeutic exercise program.

Etiology of oropharyngeal dysphagia

Transfer dysphagia involves difficulty in transferring food from the oral cavity to the esophagus and includes any pathological process from the brainstem down to the level of the cricopharyngeus muscle. It is a nonspecific symptom which is produced by an eclectic group of disorders in which the patient has trouble voluntarily transferring food from the mouth into the esophagus to initiate the involuntary phase of swallowing while protecting the airway from aspiration. The physiology of normal oropharyngeal swallowing is dependent on rapid neuromuscular coordination of structures in the oral cavity, pharynx, and larynx during a brief cessation of respiration. Swallowing frequency is greatest during eating and least during sleeping. Mean deglutition frequency is approximately 580 swallows per day. Swallowing and respiration are reciprocal functions and normally respiration halts during deglutition.

Transfer dysphagia is often associated with other phenomena such as central nervous system and cranial nerve deficits. Manifestations include drooling, speech disorders, nasal regurgitation, coughing, and choking spells. These conditions may exist singly or in combination. Factors contributing to the dysphagia are an altered mental status, depression, anorexia, fatigue, and other general illnesses, such as strokes (see Figure 5.6 for the neurological control of swallowing).

The etiologies of dysphagia have, for the sake of simplicity, been divided into neurologic causes, structural causes, and systemic causes as shown in Figure 5.7.

Neurologic causes

These neurologic conditions can involve the sensory or motor components of each stage of swallowing from the oral preparatory stage, the tongue movements, the pharyngeal swallow and the upper esophageal stage.

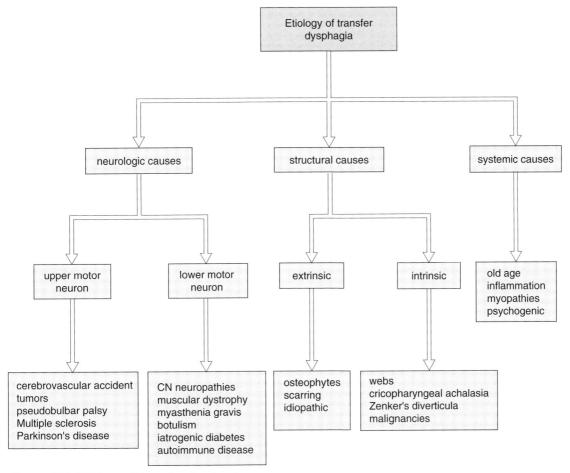

Figure 5.7 Etiology of transfer dysphagia.

Central causes

Some of the causes of central neurologic problems are discussed below.

1. Strokes involving the posterior inferior cerebellar artery or vertebrobasilar artery lead to a palsy of several cranial nerves including the trigeminal, glossopharyngeal, vagus, and accessory nerves. These result in poor velar closure and diminished laryngeal elevation. Aspiration occurs when both the superior and recurrent laryngeal nerves are involved. There is oral apraxia which involves impaired voluntary movement of the bolus in the mouth. This results in delay in bolus transfer especially in left hemispheric lesions.

2. Pseudo-bulbar palsy leads to atrophy of the pharyngeal muscles and a decrease in mucosal sensitivity.

3. Brainstem tumors affect the swallowing centers in the brainstem and impair the initiation of swallowing.

4. Neurodegenerative conditions such as Parkinson's disease, amyotrophic lateral sclerosis, multiple sclerosis and familial dysautonomia affect cognition and generally impair the oral phase of swallowing. The prevalence of Parkinson's disease is approximately 10 to 450 per 100 000 of the population and appears to be increasing as the size of the elderly population increases. It is generally slowly progressive and is usually accompanied with deficits in cognition along with dysarthria and dysphonia. Patients experience difficulties with the oral, pharyngeal, and esophageal phases of swallowing. There are problems in bolus preparation because of the tongue tremor and vallecular stasis of the bolus. Volitional cough is impaired. There is marked difficulty in switching between the voluntary and involuntary phases of swallowing. The loss of sensation the pharynx leads to poor oropharyngeal protection and an increased risk for aspiration. In fact pneumonias secondary to aspiration are the major cause of morbidity and mortality in this population.

Peripheral or lower motor neuron diseases

These conditions affect any location between the central nuclei and the myoneural junctions. They include conditions such as myasthenia gravis, and motor neuron diseases such as amytrophic lateral sclerosis and multiple sclerosis. Multiple sclerosis follows an erratic course. Myasthenia gravis has bimodal peak incidence between the ages of 21 and 30 years and then again between 61 and 70 years. There is a decrease in acetyl choline release from the neuromuscular junction leading to fatigability and hypotonicity. This is manifest by poor initiation of swallowing, decreased tongue movement, and pooling of secretions. Dysarthria and weakness of the chewing muscles are present in more than 50% of individuals. The condition is reversible with anticholinesterases.

Iatrogenic causes include surgeries in the vicinity of the pharynx that damage the pharyngeal plexus, the superior or recurrent laryngeal nerves. It also includes the neuropathies induced by thyroid surgeries, radiation damage, and skull-base operations.

Structural causes

These can be intrinsic within the lumen of the pharynx and esophagus or extrinsic and can co-exist with other sensory or motor deficits.

Extrinsic causes

Osteophytes of the cervical spine can compress the esophagus from the outside and lead to dysphagia. Congenital craniofacial syndromes include Pierre Robin's syndrome, Apert's syndrome, and Treacher Collins' syndrome. These conditions lead to nasopharyngeal and oropharyngeal obstruction secondary to abnormalities of the mandibular–hyoid relationship and a large tongue. Tracheostomies impair deglutition by preventing laryngeal elevation and by anchoring the larynx to the superficial cervical soft tissues. Other causes include malignancies of the thyroid or larynx.

Intrinsic causes

These include webs, malignancies, cricopharyngeal achalasia, and Zenker's diverticula. Webs are often associated with the Plummer–Vinson syndrome. The main symptom is dysphagia for solids.

Cricopharyngeal achalasia is associated mainly with gastroesophageal reflux or central causes such as strokes, poliomyelitis, myopathies, oculopharyngeal muscular dystrophy, post-laryngectomy, Parkinson's disease, and amyotrophic lateral sclerosis. Normally the UES should relax during swallowing. When the sphincter closes prematurely part of the bolus is trapped between the closing sphincter and the oncoming peristaltic wave. Eventually this leads to a weakening of the hypopharyngeal wall at the triangle of Killian (above the cricopharyngeus), at the triangle of Laimer (below the cricopharyngeus), or at the posterior pharyngeal wall. A protrusion of mucosa occurs leading to the formation of a Zenker's diverticulum.

Zenker's diverticula exacerbate oropharyngeal dysphagia by the pressure of the extrinsic pouch and also by the regurgitation of predigested food.

Systemic causes

This group of conditions includes problems related to the aging process, inflammatory conditions such as esophagitis, myopathies, and psychogenic conditions. In general, patients over the age of 70 develop some abnormalities of the oral and pharyngeal phases of swallowing. These difficulties may be related to the absence of dentition, poor oral hygiene, and xerostomia.

There are multiple chronic inflammatory conditions that lead to dysphagia because of indirect neurologic damage or xerostomia. Some of these include thyroiditis, scleroderma, dermatomyositis, polymyositis, systemic lupus erythematosis, sarcoidosis, amyloidosis, rheumatoid arthritis, and post-poliomyelitis.

Acute inflammatory conditions are usually of infectious etiology and include Ludwig's angina, acute tonsillitis, and peritonsillar abscesses.

Psychogenic causes can be a side effect of neuroleptics which lead to decreased salivation. Anxiety can also lead to sensations which can mimic globus and difficulties with the oral phase.

Clinical evaluation

A careful and complete case history is necessary, noting the patient's primary diagnosis, neurological status, laryngeal function, respiratory status, nutritional status, and history of any dysphagic symptoms. An evaluation of the patient's memory and cognitive status is also required.

Oral stage

Problems with this phase lead to
- drooling
- collection of food in the anterior or lateral sulci of the mouth, also called "pocketing"
- nasopharyngeal regurgitation
- increased oral transit time.

These difficulties lead to restrictions in a patient's diet and a loss of the pleasure of eating.

Pharyngeal stage

Problems with this phase lead to
- delay in pharyngeal transit time
- food collection on the weak side of the pharynx
- stasis
- otalgia in the presence of normal-appearing ears which may indicate referred pain
- aspiration and coughing. This is the most important consequence of pharyngeal swallow dysfunction. Aspiration may be caused by a delay in triggering the pharyngeal swallow mechanism, decreased laryngeal elevation, decreased laryngeal closure, cricopharyngeal dysfunction and from gastroesophageal refluxate. Also a "wet" vocal quality is indicative of penetration or aspiration.

Physical examination

At the beginning of the evaluation of a patient with dysphagia as the presenting symptom, attention should be directed to the patient's general nutritional and mental status. It is also important to determine if the patient is self-sufficient and living in an ambulatory setting or is either hospitalized or institutionalized. The aim of the physical examination in the dysphagic patient is to
1. identify whether any underlying systemic or metabolic diseases are present
2. localize, where possible, the neuroanatomic level and severity of any causative neurologic lesion
3. detect adverse sequelae such as aspiration pneumonias and nutritional deficiencies as important indicators of the severity of the dysphagia.

Neck

Palpate for the presence of an enlarged thyroid or other masses. Palpate the larynx and trachea and determine if there is a deviation from the midline, tenderness, or the inability to elevate the larynx with attempts at swallowing.

Oral cavity

Examine for palatal symmetry and check for the gag reflex. Look for masses and ulcerations in the floor of the mouth, tonsils, buccal mucosa, and the tongue. It is also important to evaluate the movement of the tongue. A bimanual palpation helps determine the extent of lesions and induration, and identify the presence of masses that may be extending into the neck.

Flexible laryngoscopy

A small telescope is passed through the nose, usually after spraying the nose with a decongestant and topical anesthetic. The endoscope is used to visualize the palate, base of tongue, valleculae, endolarynx, and piriform sinuses. Because of its small size and the absence of insufflation capacity the telescope cannot be passed into the esophageal inlet. Flexible laryngoscopy allows clear visualization of anatomic abnormalities, masses or ulcerations, and movement of the vocal folds during rest, respiration, and phonation. This relatively simple procedure is now performed almost routinely in an otolaryngology office and it can also be recorded on a videotape. The other methods of swallowing evaluation will be discussed under the next heading of diagnostic studies.

Diagnostic studies

Bedside clinical evaluation, which involves watching a patient eat and drink and determining whether or not the activity generates a cough, misses approximately 60% of patients who go on to aspirate. The following tests

help to provide a more accurate assessment of the swallowing mechanism and thereby to institute appropriate therapy. These include
1. modified barium swallow
2. functional endoscopic evaluation of swallowing (FEES)
3. functional endoscopic evaluation of swallowing with sensory testing
4. transnasal office esophagoscopy
5. manometry
6. electromyography.

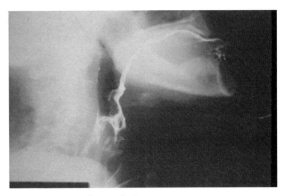

Figure 5.8 A lateral view as seen on a modified barium swallow.

Modified barium swallow

This procedure should be performed jointly by the radiologist and speech pathologist using various consistencies of barium. It is designed to evaluate the anatomy and physiology of the oral, pharyngeal, and cervical esophageal stages of deglutition and to define management strategies that will improve the safety and efficacy of swallowing in patients with oropharyngeal dysphagia. Modified barium swallow uses fluoroscopy which is a radiographic technique permitting observation of movement and providing a permanent recording of the study.

A measured amount of radiopaque barium is given in four consistencies: thin and thick liquid, puree, and solid. The patient is viewed in a normal upright feeding position and lateral and anterior projections are taken. It is important to note any residual that may be present after the initial swallow has been triggered because patients may aspirate residual material after completing the initial swallow. A lateral view is obtained followed by a posterior–anterior view. It is in this view that symmetry of the swallow and vocal-fold function can be assessed. The study is videotaped. In some institutions the esophageal phase of swallowing may also be observed. See Figures 5.8 and 5.9. This study also allows the quantification and depth of aspiration, as well as

the presence or absence of a cough reflex and the effectiveness of compensatory techniques.

A major purpose of the modified barium swallow is to identify treatment strategies that will improve the safety and efficiency of the patient's swallow. The radiographic study should not be terminated when a patient aspirates, instead a treatment strategy should be selected based on the nature of the disorder. These methods will be discussed in detail in the section on therapy (see p. 81).

Functional endoscopic evaluation of swallowing (FEES)

This procedure was originally described in 1988. It allows a complete evaluation of the pharyngeal swallowing mechanism and consists of two parts:
1. the pre-swallow assessment of the anatomy and physiology of the oropharynx and related structures
2. assessment of delivery of food and liquid to the pharynx and esophagus.
During the pre-swallow assessment, the following aspects of swallowing are examined:
• velopharyngeal closure
• lateral pharyngeal wall movement (determined with a dry swallow)

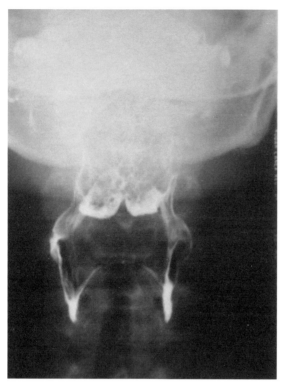

Figure 5.9 An anteroposterior (AP) view as seen on a modified barium swallow.

bolus. Generally one starts with thick liquids (nectar consistency) and moves onto purees, semisolids, and finally thin liquids which are the hardest to handle (See Figure 5.10). The following are examined:

- initiation of the swallow; look for lingual velar leakage and overflow spillage before the patient is asked to swallow
- the actual swallow; this is the "white-out" phase–look for residue in the laryngeal vestibule, vocal cords, subglottis, and trachea; ask the patient to cough to clear any aspirated material
- after the swallow maintain the endoscopy to recheck and then give a second bolus; look for esophageal regurgitation.

Advantages of FEES:

- it can be combined with therapeutic interventions
- it allows the observation of normal eating and drinking behaviors, e.g. alterations in bolus size, postural changes, and biofeedback
- it determines the risk of aspiration
- there is no exposure to radiation and it can therefore be repeated easily without risk.

- base of tongue, vallecula, and piriform sinuses for movement and residual material
- laryngeal airway protection ability
- handling of normal secretions – pharyngeal squeeze.

It is important to look at laryngeal movement during respiration, sniffing, and phonation, and to determine how the vocal folds work during coughing and breath-holding. The site and amount of pooling should also be determined.

During assessment of the swallow the nasopharyngoscope is positioned above the epiglottis and a panoramic view of the larynx is obtained. Between swallows the endoscope is lowered into the larynx to evaluate for penetration and aspiration. Various consistencies of foods incorporating a food dye are then used to easily identify the course taken by the

Functional endoscopic evaluation of swallowing with sensory testing

This method of evaluating both the sensory and motor components of swallowing can be performed at the bedside or in the office. It combines both the established endoscopic evaluation of swallowing with a technique that determines laryngopharyngeal sensory discrimination by endoscopically delivering air-pulse stimuli to the mucosa innervated by the superior laryngeal nerve. After the delivery of a pulse of air, transient vocal-fold closure (also known as the laryngeal adductor reflex) is determined by direct visualization on a video monitor receiving a real-time image from the fiberoptic telescope. Unrecognized sensory deficits in the laryngopharynx can lead to dysphagia and aspiration based on the premise that if food and secretions in the laryngopharynx cannot be felt, protective reflexes cannot be initiated and secretions and debris will descend into both the esophagus and tracheobronchial tree. Functional endoscopic evaluation of swallowing with sensory testing allows the clinician additional objective measures to help guide the behavioral and dietary management of patients and reduce their risk of aspiration.

Office-based endoscopy

Advances in fiberoptic and videoendoscopic technology have made the diagnosis of upper aerodigestive tract pathology easier to perform both from a technical and a practice-efficiency perspective. The use of transnasal esophagoscopy is a relatively new method which allows the passage of a small flexible endoscope of approximately 5 mm diameter beyond the cricopharyngeus into the cervical esophagus. The scope can then be passed through the thoracic esophagus to the gastroesophageal junction. Mucosal irregularities, masses, or areas of narrowing are noted. Most patients in whom these procedures have been performed have tolerated it very well. It is recommended in patients who have had a previous non-contributory examination of the oropharynx and hypopharynx for the evaluation of dysphagia.

Manometry

The use of esophageal manometry to diagnose motility disorders of the esophagus is widely accepted; however, the utility of pharyngeal and UES assessment with circumferentially sensing transducers that accurately measure pressure and coordination sequences during swallowing is relatively new. Manometric investigation of the UES and the cricopharyngeus and pharynx can now be performed in specialized swallowing centers.

For patients suffering from oropharyngeal dysphagia, a barium swallow study and manometry are complimentary. Their combined use permits an enhanced understanding of the pathophysiologic processes that are causing the patient's symptoms. Abnormalities have been noted in diseases such as Parkinson's disease, oculopharyngeal muscular dystrophy, achalasia, and scleroderma. Pharyngeal and UES manometry also help in evaluating patients who are candidates for a myotomy or dilatation, as it can help identify patients with a potentially good outcome.

Electromyography

This method is useful in studying the pharyngeal phase of swallowing. Electromyography of the cricopharyngeus muscle and the laryngeal muscles is useful primarily for the evaluation of neurologic disorders affecting the swallowing mechanism. It can be performed with needle electrodes, hooked wire electrodes, or with surface electrodes. It provides information about specific groups of muscles. Four patterns of response with different diagnostic or prognostic interpretations are obtained – normal, denervation, reinnervation and central. The patterns of response offer the possibility of determining the existence of lesions of the recurrent and superior laryngeal nerves. The physiologic age of injury and prognosis after an injury can also be obtained. Alone electromyography is of limited value but in conjunction with other tests it can provide significant information that is useful for the diagnosis, prognosis, and therapy of swallowing disorders.

Management of oropharyngeal dysphagia

The treatment of transfer dysphagia is dependent on the etiology and magnitude of the dysphagia. When a patient is first

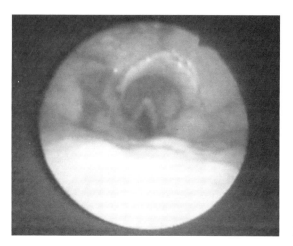

Figure 5.10 An endoscopic view as seen during the FEES procedure. Pooling is observed at the piriform sinuses. (See p. xvii for color)

identified with dysphagia the authors recommend a multidisciplinary approach to the evaluation and management of this condition. For the majority of patients dysphagia is one of the most disabling and debilitating of conditions. Treatment of underlying disorders when present is usually with medications (e.g. for Parkinson's disease and myasthenia gravis) and possibly with surgery (e.g for vocal cord paralysis). The treatment strategies designed to specifically address the dysphagia are discussed below.

Conservative management

Postural therapy

This form of therapy may change pharyngeal dimensions or the gravitational flow of food through the oral cavity and pharynx thereby reducing the risk of aspiration and increasing the amount of material entering the esophagus. It is important to understand the physiological changes that each particular postural change produces. These therapeutic maneuvers are generally under the care of a swallowing therapist. They include the following:

1. Head tilting forward or chin tuck. This pushes the anterior wall of the pharynx posteriorly, significantly narrowing the airway entrance and pushing the tongue base and epiglottis farther backward toward the posterior pharyngeal wall. In some patients the chin-tuck posture results in a widened vallecular space as the tongue falls forward and the epiglottis falls somewhat backward. This posture is often helpful for the patient with a delayed swallow, reduced laryngeal closure, and reduced tongue-base retraction.

2. Head tilting backward. This facilitates gravitational drainage of food out of the oral cavity and thus improves the speed of the oral transit time and is used in patients with poor tongue control or whose tongue has been partially resected.

3. Mendelson's manuever. This method is designed to maintain the larynx at its maximally elevated position by having the patient swallow and hold the larynx up. It enhances airway protection by allowing opening of the UES with easier passage of the bolus.

4. Supraglottic swallow. This method involves hypercontraction of the supraglottic structures while holding the breath and coughing after the swallow. It provides improved airway protection. The patient must be alert, relatively relaxed, and able to follow simple directions.

5. Extended supraglottic swallow. This is used with those patients who have severe reductions in tongue mobility or tongue bulk because of surgical procedures and with little or no oral transit. After the supraglottic swallow the patient performs a valsalva and bears down during the time when they are holding their breath. This method is designed to close the entrance to the airway voluntarily by tilting the arytenoid cartilage anteriorly to the base of the epiglottis before and during the swallow. It is helpful in patients after a supraglottic laryngectomy and involves extra effort to increase the anterior arytenoid tilt.

These conservative measures are usually monitored with endoscopic swallowing evaluations periodically. They can be used in combination with one another. They are mainly compensatory strategies and do not alter the patient's physiologic capacity or neuromuscular control.

Diet consistency strategies

These are designed to promote easier transfer of the bolus and to reduce the risk of aspiration. The patient may be recommended to eat or drink mechanical soft, puree, honey thick liquids and/or nectar liquids.

Behavior modification

1. Timing of meals. This is important as timing meals with periods of optimal alertness makes the process of feeding easier with greater compliance on the part of the patient.
2. Supervision of a patient if they are self-feeding.
3. Assistance in cases of debilitated patients or those with neurological deficits.
4. Biofeedback. This method allows visual or proprioceptive cues to be used to educate the patient in manuevers that will assist in feeding and decrease the risk of aspiration. The use of videolaryngoscopy often helps to show the patient how aspiration occurs and how postural and other methods assist in improving swallowing.

Oropharyngeal exercises

These are recommended by the speech language pathologist. These include tactile kinesthetic approaches, thermal stimulation, pressure application, and oral-muscle exercises. Cold stimulation has been shown to be most effective in eliciting a swallow. The purpose of thermal stimulation is to increase sensory awareness in the oral cavity prior to

the swallow and to decrease any delay between the oral and pharyngeal swallow. A laryngeal mirror dipped in iced water is rubbed on the faucial arches four to five times in a rapid fashion. The patient is then asked to swallow saliva or a small amount of thickened cold liquid. The result is a decrease in the timing of the initiation of the swallow reflex.

Surgical therapy

Vocal cord medialization

This technique is very helpful for patients with a paralyzed vocal cord. It helps in decreasing the risk of aspiration by allowing the patient to generate a strong cough reflex to clear any aspirated material from the tracheobronchial tree. It can be performed by injecting a variety of materials into the paralyzed vocal cord and thereby augmenting the bulk of the cord and allowing glottic closure. The materials injected include collagen, fat, and micronized dermis amongst others. Most of these materials are absorbable over a period of time. The other method of medializing a paralyzed vocal cord is by the placement of an implant in a window created in the thyroid cartilage. The implants can be made of soft silastic, titanium, silicone, or GORE-TEX®. These implants are generally long lasting. The procedure takes longer than the injection method and is recommended for patients with a large glottic gap or in those with long-standing paralysis with no chance of recovery of function.

Chemical myotomy

Botulinum toxin is a potent neurotoxin that blocks release of acetyl choline at the neuromuscular junction. Weakness is related to the number of motor end plates paralyzed, which is a dose-related phenomenon. Using a percutaneous technique with electromyographic guidance botulinum toxin is injected into the cricopharyngeus muscle to relieve spasm. The cricopharyngeus muscle is active at rest and relatively silent during a swallow. Once the correct position of the needle electrode is ascertained the toxin is injected. Both sides are generally injected. This method also serves as a test to determine if a myotomy of the cricopharyngeus will help with the treatment of dysphagia. In patients who are poor operative risks, botulinum toxin injections alone may serve as therapy.

Cricopharyngeal myotomy

This procedure is recommended in patients who have incomplete relaxation of the UES with or without a Zenker's diverticulum. It is often seen in patients with neuromuscular disorders (e.g. amyotrophic lateral sclerosis, multiple sclerosis and cerebrovascular accidents). It is contraindicated in patients with severe gastroesophageal reflux. The procedure involves a myotomy and resection of about 3 cm of the cricopharyngeal muscle. The overall success rate of this procedure is 80% in properly selected cases.

Cricopharyngeal dilatation

This is performed in patients with a stricture or a web at the level of the cricopharyngeus muscle. It is performed with a large-bore dilator and carries a risk of esophageal perforation.

Tracheostomy

Although the presence of a tracheostomy does not preclude aspiration it allows patients with significant aspiration into the tracheobronchial tree to get aggressive pulmonary toilet thereby decreasing the risk of aspiration pneumonias.

Promotion of alimentation

Alternative forms of nutrition are necessary in patients who cannot meet their nutritional needs in those at very high risk of aspiration. These modes of nutrition can be enteral or parenteral.

Enteral

This allows liquid nutrients to be given via a nasogastric or gastrostomy tube. In patients where there is significant risk of gastroesophageal reflux or disease affecting the stomach, nutrition can also be given via a J-tube directly into the jejunum.

Parenteral

In patients where there is a problem with absorption through the gastrointestinal tract nutrition is given directly into the bloodstream. This can be via a peripheral line (peripheral parenteral nutrition) or a central line (total parenteral nutrition).

Conclusion

Oropharyngeal or transfer dysphagia requires a multidisciplinary approach to its diagnosis and subsequent management. The goal of treatment is generally empiric and is to provide a safe swallow and provide the individual with adequate nutrition. The newer diagnostic methods being used are non-invasive, they carry less risk of radiation exposure, and allow biofeedback to be used in therapy.

Further reading

Aviv JE, Takoudes TG, Guoguang MA, Close LG. Office-based esophagoscopy: a preliminary report. *Otolaryngol. Head Neck Surg* 2001; 125(3): 170–175.

Broniatowski M, Sonies BC, Rubin JS, *et al*. Current evaluation and treatment of patients with swallowing disorders. *Otolaryngol Head Neck Surg* 1999; 120(4): 464–473.

Castell JA, Castell DO. Upper esophageal sphincter and pharyngeal function and oropharyngeal (transfer) dysphagia. *Gastro Clin N Amer* 1996; 25(1): 35–50.

Langmore SE, McCulloch TM. *Examination of the Pharynx and Larynx and Endoscopic Examination of Pharyngeal Swallowing. Deglutition and its disorders*. A. Perlman, K. Schultz (eds), Singular Press, San Diego, 1996.

Logemann JA. *Evaluation and Treatment of Swallowing Disorders*. Pro-ed., Austin, TX, 1983.

Logemann JA. Swallowing physiology and pathophysiology. *Otolaryngol Clin N Am* 1988; 21(4): 613–623.

Chapter 6

Rings, Webs, Stenoses, and Diverticula of the Esophagus

Faten N. Aberra and David A. Katzka

Introduction

There are many anatomic abnormalities of the esophagus that may be congenital or acquired in origin. This chapter will specifically address esophageal rings, webs, stenoses, and diverticula. Muscular and mucosal esophageal rings will be described. Types of benign and malignant stenoses will be described. Pharyngoesophageal diverticula, midesophageal diverticula, epiphrenic diverticula, and intramural pseudodiverticulosis will be defined. Information will be provided on the underlying etiology, clinical manifestions, diagnostic tests, and treatment options for these abnormalities.

Esophageal rings

There are three types of esophageal rings named A, B, and C. All are located in the esophageal vestibule, a region that normally appears slightly distended and which is located proximal to the gastroesophageal junction. A-type esophageal rings are muscular in origin. B-type rings are mucosal in origin, and C-type rings are a nonpathologic radiographic anomaly caused by the diaphragm indenting on the esophagus; they are never symptomatic.

Muscular rings

The muscular esophageal ring, or A ring, is located 1.5 cm proximal to the squamocolumnar junction. The ring is comprised of hypertrophied or hypertonic muscle covered with normal squamous epithelium. The exact etiology of muscular rings is not known, but there appears to be an association with motility disorders, GERD, and hiatal hernias. The most common symptom associated with muscular rings is intermittent dysphagia, although most patients with muscular rings are asymptomatic.

Diagnosis

Barium esophagram depicts muscular rings as smooth, symmetrical narrowings that are broader than mucosal rings longitudinally and during full distension of the esophagus findings of the ring may disappear. Esophageal manometry may reveal a hypertensive LES that correlates with the location of the ring by barium esophagram.

Treatment

If patients are symptomatic they are treated. Rings may be treated with passage of 16.5 to 20 mm (50–60 Fr) Maloney dilators. Repeat treatment may be needed over time. Botulinum toxin-A has also been shown to help in patients who have underlying motility disorders.

Mucosal rings

The mucosal esophageal ring, or B ring, also known as Schatzki ring, is located at the level of the squamocolumnar–mucosal junction. The ring is comprised of mucosa and submucosa. The mucosal epithelium on the proximal side of the ring is squamous and on the distal side of the ring it may be either columnar or several millimeters of squamous then columnar.

As in muscular rings most mucosal rings are asymptomatic. Rings greater than 20 mm in luminal diameter rarely cause symptoms. Symptoms usually occur when the luminal diameter is less than 13 mm. Symptomatic patients are commonly over 40 years of age

and the most common symptom is intermittent solid-food dysphagia.

The etiology of the B ring is not known, although some evidence suggests that gastroesophageal reflux may cause B-type rings.

Diagnosis

By barium esophagram mucosal rings appear as a thin transverse ridge above the hiatus of the gastroesophageal junction. Unlike muscular rings, mucosal rings are best seen with distension of the gastroesophageal region. Indeed, without proper radiologic technique, subtle rings can easily be missed. Valsalva maneuver during esophagram may help in detecting the ring. A 13 mm barium tablet or marshmallow bolus given to a patient while standing increases the sensitivity of detection of the ring. Although they are more advanced techniques, double-contrast barium esophagram and endoscopy are not as sensitive as single-contrast barium esophagram with or without barium tablet or marshmallow bolus in determining mucosal rings.

Treatment

Treatment of symptomatic rings should include trial of passage of a 16.5 to 20 mm (50–60 Fr) Maloney dilator. Repeat treatment may be needed over time. If dilation fails then electrocautery incision using needle knife papillotome has been reported as a safe and effective technique. Simple obliteration with a biopsy forceps may also be useful. There is also a question of whether patients with recurrent ring formation should be studied and treated for reflux disease.

Esophageal webs

Esophageal webs are thin, transverse membranes of squamous epithelium located in the upper and midesophagus usually a few centimeters away from the cricopharyngeus. Webs are usually on the anterior surface of the esophagus and rarely involve the entire circumference. The prevalence of webs in patients presenting with dysphagia ranges from 5% to 15% and the prevalence increases with age. Although the etiology of esophageal webs is unknown, it is believed that most webs are remnants of incomplete replacement of the esophageal columnar epithelium during the early embryonic stage. Midesophageal webs may be single or multiple and are believed to be congenital in origin. Some recent literature also supports a role for reflux disease in the formation of webs.

The association of iron deficiency and esophageal webs was first noted by laryngologists Patterson and Kelly and gastroenterologists Plummer and Vinson. The syndrome of esophageal webs, iron-deficiency anemia, glossitis, koilonychia, and increased risk for pharyngeal and cervical esophageal cancer has been termed both the Plummer–Vinson syndrome and the Patterson–Kelly syndrome. There have been no studies proving the causative role of iron deficiency and webs. Cervical webs have been associated with heterotopic gastric tissue. During embryonic development columnar epithelium in the upper esophagus may not be entirely replaced by pseudo-stratified squamous epithelium resulting in heterotopic islands of gastric mucosa. The formation of the webs is believed to be a result of chronic injury from local acid production by oxyntic cells in the heterotopic gastric tissue. Other diseases associated with webs include thyroid disease, esophageal duplication cyst and Zenker's diverticula, chronic graft-versus-host disease after allogenic bone marrow transplantation, blistering skin diseases (cicatricial pemphigoid, mucous-membrane pemphigoid, and epidermolysis bullosa), psoriasis, idiopathic eosinophilic esophagitis, Stevens–Johnson syndrome, radiation, and caustic injury; see Box 6.1.

Diagnosis

Patients with esophageal webs are usually asymptomatic, but when symptoms are present the most common one is solid-food dysphagia followed by nasopharyngeal reflux and/or aspiration. Barium studies are the most sensitive diagnositic tests for webs. Video-radiography with lateral and anteroposterior views should be taken during the study. If a barium swallow is completed, then a careful evaluation of the postcricoid area is required. Diagnosing esophageal webs by upper endoscopy is more difficult for several reasons. Webs are easily missed because of their proximal location or they may be pierced and not seen if the scope is advanced quickly and without complete visualization into the esophagus. Sometimes after resistance to passage of the scope, finding blood in the proximal esophagus may indicate unexpected web rupture. The advantage of endoscopy is that heterotopic gastric tissue may be observed. The differential diagnosis of esophageal webs by endoscopic findings include inflammatory stenosis, postcricoid carcinoma, and postcricoid impression due to ventral venous plexus.

Box 6.1 Diseases associated with esophageal webs

Congenital conditions
Plummer–Vinson syndrome
Heterotopic gastric tissue
Thyroid disease
Esophageal duplication cysts
Zenker's diverticulum
Chronic graft-versus-host disease
Cicatricial pemphigoid
Epidermolysis bullosa
Psoriasis
Idiopathic eosinophilic esophagitis
Stevens–Johnson syndrome
Radiation injury
Caustic injury

Treatment

Treatment is based on symptoms. Mild symptoms associated with small webs can be treated with changes in dietary habits, such as cutting and chewing food more carefully and eating more slowly. If this is not sufficient, dilation should be performed by passage of an endoscope, bougie, or balloon, particularly in patients with more persistent and/or significant luminal compromise. There have been reports of neodymium:yttrium–aluminum–garnet laser therapy used successfully for treatment of webs and can be considered in patients refractory to dilation. Surgical therapy should only be considered in cases refractory to dilation which is rare or cases that are associated with Zenker's diverticulum.

Stenoses

Obstruction of the esophagus can be categorized as extrinsic or intrinsic. Extrinsic causes of esophageal obstruction in the cervical region include enlarged thyroid or parathyroid glands, tumors, cervical adenopathy, osteophytes, and an anteriorly herniatied disc in the cervical spine. In the thorax extrinsic esophageal stenoses are caused by mediastinal adenopathy or tumor, a right aortic arch, aortic aneurysm, a tortuous aorta, aberrant subclavian artery, pericardial effusion, an enlarged left atrium, or a lung tumor. Intrinsic stenoses of the esophagus are categorized as benign or malignant. See Box 6.2 for differential diagnoses of esophageal strictures.

Benign strictures

Peptic strictures

The most common esophageal stricture is related to GERD. Long-standing untreated

Box 6.2 Differential diagnosis of esophageal strictures

Caustic ingestion
Congenital esophageal stenosis
Crohn's disease
Eosinophilic esophagitis
Epidermolysis bullosa
Esophageal atresia
Graft-versus-host disease
Infections
  monilia
  tuberculosis
  typhoid
  herpes simplex
  cytomegalovirus
Intramural pseudodiverticulosis
Malignancy
Medications
  alendronate
  clindamycin
  cromolyn sodium
  ferrous sulfate
  isotretinoin
  NSAIDS
  phenytoin
  potassium chloride and citrate
  quinidine
  sodium valproate
  tetracycline
  vitamin C
Postoperative
Radiation
Sclerotherapy

esophagitis from GERD may lead to esophageal stricture formation, also known as peptic stricture, and is estimated to occur in 7% to 23% of patients with chronic, untreated, reflux esophagitis. Peptic strictures are ten times more common in Caucasians than in African Americans or Asians. They are commonly found in patients with Barrett's esophagus.

Peptic strictures usually form at the squamo-columnar junction and may be located more proximally in patients with Barrett's esophagus. The length of these strictures is usually less than 1 cm, but it can occasionally extend to 8 cm. For strictures longer than 3 to 4 cm, predisposing conditions such as Zollinger–Ellison syndrome, superimposed pill esophagitis, or prolonged nasogastric intubation should be considered. Histopathology reveals that with increasing severity of esophagitis, inflammation extends deeper into the wall of the esophagus with stricture formation resulting from transmural inflammation.

The most common presenting symptom is dysphagia, usually for solids, but may progress to include liquids. When patients first present dysphagia is usually present for 4 to 6 years prior. Up to 75% will also have a history of heartburn. Heartburn symptoms decline with more severe stricture obstruction. Patients may also present with atypical symptoms such as chronic cough and asthma from aspiration and reflex bronchoconstriction respectively. Chest pain may result from esophagitis, esophageal spasm or food impaction at the level of the stricture.

Diagnosis Diagnosis is best made with barium esophagography as the initial study since it provides information about the location, diameter, and length of the stricture. Techniques such as rapid swallowing, Valsalva maneuver, use of 13 mm tablets or food aid in the identification of the stricture site. Endoscopy is useful in defining the extent and etiology of a stricture. The endoscopic appearance is a smooth stenosis, usually in the distal esophagus, that fails to open with air insufflation, with esophagitis seen in half the cases. Biopsies of the stricture should be taken from the proximal edge and blindly from the depths of the stricture. One should be cautioned that strictures with a luminal diameter of 13 mm or greater may be missed especially with use of a thin endoscope or minimal conscious sedation.

Treatment The cornerstone of therapy involves acid suppression with proton pump inhibitors and dilation of the stricture. The use of proton pump inhibitors in randomized controlled trials starting at doses of omeprazole 20 mg a day and lansoprazole 30 mg a day have shown to decrease frequency of dilation. There are several types of bougienage. Two types of dilators may be used: balloon and rigid-type dilators; see Tables 6.1 and 6.2.

The "rules of threes" should be followed when dilating peptic strictures. That is to pass no more than three consecutive dilators that meet moderate resistance during a single dilating session. Most strictures that an endoscope can pass through can be dilated without fluoroscopic guidance. Tight, complicated strictures should be dilated under fluoroscopic guidance or with a through-the-scope balloon.

In the past one-third to one-half of patients have required long-term, repeat dilations with the peak requirement for dilation in the first year. Hopefully with the use of proton pump inhibitors this has lessened. The length and diameter of the stricture do not determine the need for repeat dilation. Esophageal perforation rates for dilation of peptic strictures for all types of dilators is about 0.25%. The perforation rates for wire-guided dilators alone range from 0.4% to 0.6%. Reduction of esophageal perforation may occur if the anatomy of the esophagus and the stricture is checked by endoscopy and barium esophagram prior to dilation, if the dilation is performed slowly, and if fluoroscopy is issued in initial dilations and when dilating complex strictures.

Indications for surgery are a non-dilatable stricture, frequent stricture recurrence after dilation, and failure to control esophagitis and recurrent stricture formation on maximal medical therapy. Surgical options for peptic stricture and GERD include stricturoplasty and fundoplication. Contraindications to performing a fundoplication are a non-dilatable stricture, a prior partial gastrectomy, and severe esophageal shortening. Patients with

Table 6.1 Esophageal dilators

Dilators	Indication	Advantages
Mercury Bougies	Short strictures that are not angulated or tortuous.	Fluoroscopy not required. Performed in an outpatient setting.
Guidewire-directed	Long, tight or angulated strictures.	Flexible and easier to pass through the mouth and pharynx.
Polyethylene balloons	Long, tight, or angulated strictures.	Performed at time of endoscopy. Fluoroscopy is not required. Easy to use.

severe esophagal shortening may require gastroplasty (Collis procedure) and fundoplication or a less preferred esophagoplasty (Thal procedure) that does not prevent reflux and has a higher mortality. Esophagoplasty involves making a longitudinal, full-thickness incision in the stricture which is then covered with a gastric serosal patch. Patients with a prior history of gastric resection may benefit from a Roux-en-Y for bile acid diversion. Patients with irreversible damage to the esophagus may require esophagectomy with reconstruction. Patients may require postsurgical dilation but less frequently than those medically treated. It is not clear whether intralesional steroid therapy is helpful in the management of peptic strictures.

Caustic injury

Chronic esophageal stricture formation is common after caustic injury. These strictures are characteristically long and rigid and may involve any part of the esophagus as well as the stomach. They typically require repeated dilations, often complicated by perforation. Occasionally surgery with intestinal interposition is needed.

Radiation esophagitis

Exposure of the esophagus to radiation may induce esophagitis, injuring the epithelium and submucosal endothelium. Strictures that form as a result of radiation-induced esophagitis occur months to decades after exposure; they may vary from short to long strictures. Dilation is the treatment of choice.

Pill esophagitis

Several medications have been implicated in inducing pill esophagitis (see Box 6.2). In some cases, this may lead to acute stricture formation in the mid- or distal esophagus. Chronic strictures from pill-induced injury are uncommon. Usually, if a stricture is found, the esophagitis is a result of a pill lodging in the stricture site.

Infections

There have been reports of stricture in patients with candida esophagitis, CMV esophagitis, *Mycobacterium tuberculosis* infections, and, rarely, in idiopathic esophageal ulcers in primary HIV infection.

Table 6.2 Type and description of dilators

Dilators	Description	Sizes
Mercury Bougies		
Hurst	Mercury-filled blunt tip.	3–20 mm (10–60 Fr)
Maloney	Mercury-filled tapered tip.	3–20 mm (10–60 Fr)
Guidewire-directed		
Jackson-Plummer; Eder Puestow	Guidewire-directed that have been replaced.	
Savory-Gillard	Hollow-core polyvinyl dilator with a tapered tip, radiopaque markings for use with fluoroscopy, guidewire-directed.	5–20 mm (15–60 Fr)
American	Similar to Savory but dilator is impregnated with barium and has shorter tapered tip.	7–20 mm (21–60 Fr)
Celestin	Neoplex stepped diameter dilators, consists of two tapered dilators, guidewire-directed.	12 mm maximum and 18 mm maximum
Keymed advanced dilator	Three spindle-shaped silicone bougies on stainless-steel shafts.	
Polyethylene balloons		
Through-the-scope; guidewire facilitated	Graded and fixed diameter balloons that also vary in length.	4–40 mm diameter (12–120 Fr)
Hybrid through-the-scope guidewire		100–200 cm length

Other benign inflammatory induced strictures

Other inflammatory diseases, excluding infections affecting the esophagus, may occasionally lead to formation of strictures. Many of these diseases have extragastrointestinal manifestations that aid in determining a diagnosis.

Eosinophilic esophagitis can be a rare manifestation of eosinophilic gastroenteritis syndrome or it may occur alone. It is characterized by gastrointestinal symptoms, peripheral eosinophilia (although this may be absent), and infiltration of the esophageal tissue by mature eosinophils. Eosinophilic esophagitis is frequently associated with allergic disorders or specific food intolerance. Strictures that may form are usually proximal in location and pseudomembrane formation may be seen proximal to the stricture. Intraepithelial esophageal eosinophils greater in number than 20 per high-powered field have been used as a diagnostic criterion. Treatment of strictures is usually successful with dilation. Steroids and/or food-elimination diets may be considered post-dilation for patients with persistent symptoms.

Epidermolysis bullosa and cicatricial pemphigoid (also known as benign mucous membrane pemphigoid) are blistering dermatologic diseases. Cicatricial pemphigoid primarily causes strictures in the cervical esophagus, but may also in the mid and lower esophagus. Epidermolysis bullosa tends to form multiple strictures associated with esophageal shortening and motility abnormalities located in the upper esophageal sphincter, carina, and distal esophagus. Rarely lichen planus, another skin disease, may also cause esophageal strictures. Sarcoidosis, Crohn's disease, Behçet's syndrome, and graft-versus-host disease are other systemic inflammatory disorders resulting in strictures. Endoscopy is indicated in all the above diagnoses except for epidermolysis bullosa because of the risk of trauma bullae formation. Barium esophagram is the test of choice in epidermolysis bullosa.

Congenital esophageal stenosis

Congenital esophageal stenosis, a rare disease, is caused when tracheobronchial remnants, arising from defective separation of the embryologic respiratory tract, form the primitive foregut or abnormal esophageal wall muscle. Patients usually are diagnosed in infancy and childhood, but may occasionally present in adulthood. Patients usually have a history of long-standing dysphagia to solids and may have a history of food impaction. Misdiagnosis as peptic stricture or esophageal webs is common. Strictures are seen in the upper, mid-, or distal esophagus and tend to be long with normal overlying mucosa. By double-contrast barium esophagram the esophagus tapers with concentric narrowing and transverse ring-like indentations may be seen in the area of narrowing. In addition to endoscopy confirming normal mucosa, endoscopic ultrasound is recommended to exclude secondary causes of esophageal stenosis. Therapy involves vigorous dilation that tends to cause chest pain.

Malignant (tumor) strictures

Several types of tumors may lead to esophageal stenosis. Esophageal malignant tumors include adenocarcinoma, squamous cell carcinoma, adenocanthoma/adenosquamous carcinomas, adenoid cystic carcinoma, mucoepidermoid carcinoma, melanoma, small cell carcinoma, and choriocarcinoma. Benign non-epithelial tumors include leiomyomas and lymphangiomas. Malignant non-epithelial tumors include leiomyosarcoma and metastatic carcinoma.

Diverticula

Esophageal diverticula can be divided anatomically into four categories: pharyngoesophageal diverticula, midesophageal diverticula, epiphrenic diverticula, and intramural pseudodiverticulosis. Pathophysiologically, they can also be divided based on formation due to traction and pulsion. Most diverticula are due to pulsion from lack of a muscular coat of the esophageal wall in that region. The following description of esophageal diverticula will be based on anatomic location, since this classification scheme is most commonly used.

Pharyngoesophageal diverticula

The main type of pharyngoesophageal diverticulum is a Zenker's diverticulum. This pulsion diverticulum is formed by protrusion of posterior hypopharyngeal mucosa between the oblique fibers of the inferior pharyngeal constrictor and transverse fibers of the cricopharyngeus; this region is also referred to Killian's triangle, proximal to the esophagus above the UES. It was previously believed that UES discoordination was a condition that leads to Zenker's diverticulum formation. Studies have shown that this is not true and that reduced UES compliance may lead to high hypopharyngeal pressures. High hypopharyngeal pressures in combination with an area of weakness in the posterior hypopharyngeal wall leads to formation of the diverticulum.

The prevalence of Zenker's diverticulum increases with age and reaches 50% in the seventh and eighth decades of life. Most patients are asymptomatic and are diagnosed by chance during radiologic evaluation. Symptoms, if present, tend to be based on the severity of the diverticulum and UES dysfunction. Early in the disease patients may complain of a sensation of sticking in the throat or of vague irritation, intermittent cough, excessive salivation, and intermittent dysphagia to solids. As the diverticulum becomes larger patients may complain of more frequent dysphagia to solids, regurgitation of food, gurgling sounds upon swallowing, nocturnal coughing, and halitosis. Patients may inadvertently learn techniques to resolve symptoms such as pressing on the neck, coughing, or clearing the throat. Rarely, the diverticulum may become so large to cause obstruction and bulging in the left side of the neck. Other complications are rare and include massive bleeding, tracheoesophageal fistula, and possibly increased risk for esophageal carcinoma, usually squamous cell.

Diagnosis

The diagnostic test of choice is barium esophagram. The diverticulum can be seen posteriorly with barium falling into the pouch, although a careful evaluation of the pharyngeal phase with lateral and oblique views should be done so that small diverticula are not missed. Another diverticulum that may be confused with Zenker's diverticulum is the Killian–Jamieson diverticulum which occurs below the UES on the lateral wall and tends to be asymptomatic. Endoscopy is not recommended for diagnosis because of the risk of penetrating the diverticulum leading to perforation, but may be needed if surgery is required to exclude malignancy.

Treatment

Symptomatic diverticula require treatment and the only effective therapy is surgery. Surgical options include diverticulopexy or, diverticulectomy, in association with cricopharyngeal myotomy, which may be done individually or in combination. Endoscopic techniques are available and involve creating a communication, either by incision or laser therapy, through the septum that divides the esophageal lumen and diverticulum.

Midesophageal diverticula

Diverticula in this location are believed to arise from motility disorders and in the past were believed to form from traction of the esophagus from mediastinal inflammation resulting in all layers of the esophagus creating an outpouching. Midesophageal diverticula are found in both young and older adults.

These diverticula tend to be small and thus are rarely symptomatic. There have been reports of patients complaining of chest pain and dysphagia, but many of these patients had motility disorders that could account for the symptoms. Complications are rare and are similar to that of Zenker's diverticulum and include spontaneous rupture, exsanguinations, aspiration, fistula formation, and carcinoma.

Diagnosis

Most diverticula are found by chance in barium esophagram. They may appear singly or multiply and come in various sizes. By endoscopy, they may appear wide mouthed. If diverticula are seen a motility disorder should be considered.

Treatment

Treatment is rarely needed, but if required diverticulectomy with or without myotomy is recommended.

Epiphrenic diverticula

Diverticula that occur in the distal 3 to 4 cm of the esophagus are referred to as epiphrenic. They usually occur as a result of a motility disorder, most likely achalasia or diffuse esophageal spasm. Epiphrenic diverticula occur at all ages. Symptoms, unlike other types of esophageal diverticula, usually result from the associated motility disorder, unless the diverticulum is large. Patients may present with chest pain and regurgitation. Complications are similar to that of midesophageal diverticula.

Diagnosis

As in the other esophageal diverticula, barium esophagram is the diagnostic test of choice. If this form of diverticulum is suspected then manometry should be completed. If complications are suspected endoscopy is a useful evaluative tool.

Treatment

As long as the diverticulum is small, the goal should be treating the underlying motility disorder to prevent further enlargement of the diverticulum, usually requiring UES myotomy. Dilation is contraindicated because of the risk of perforation of the diverticulum. If patients are symptomatic with a large diverticulum, then diverticulotomy is often required at the time of myotomy.

Intramural pseudodiverticulosis

Dilation of the excretory ducts, possibly resulting from blockage by inflammatory debris of the submucosal esophageal glands, may lead to formation of pseudodiverticulosis. The underlying pathophysiology is unclear. Patients are primarily elderly, usually in their sixth and seventh decades. Most patients have symptoms of chronic dysphagia to solids. Stricture formation, usually distal to the pseudodiverticulosis, has been seen in 70% to 90% of patients. Candida esophagitis has been seen in 50% of cases, although the correlation between candida and pseudodiverticulosis has not been established.

Diagnosis

Double-constrast barium esophagram is the test of choice for diagnosis since pseudodiverticula are small and may go unrecognized by endoscopy. Diffuse or segmental involvement may be present.

Treatment

Dilation is the treatment of choice since strictures commonly coexist with pseudodiverticula; it is usually successful in relieving symptoms. Repeat dilations may be required in some patients.

Further reading

Boyce GA, Boyce HW. Esophagus: anatomy and structural anomalies. In Yamada T, Alpers DH, Laine L, *et al.* (eds) *Textbook of Gastroentorology* vol. 1, 3rd edn, Philadelphia, PA: Lippincott Williams & Wilkins; 1999.

Cook IJ, Gabb M, Panagopoulos V, *et al.* Pharyngeal (Zenker's) diverticulum is a disorder of upper esophageal sphincter opening. *Gastroenterology* 1992; 03: 229–235.

Hoffman RM, Jaffe PE. Plummer–Vinson syndrome: case report and literature review. *Arch Intern Med* 1995; 155: 2008–2011.

Jerome-Zapadka KM, Clarke MR, Sekas G. Recurrent upper esophageal webs in association with heterotopic gastric mucosa: case report and literature review. *Am J Gastroenterol* 1994; 89: 421–424.

Katzka DA, Levine MS, Ginsberg GG, *et al.* Congenital esophageal stenosis in adults. *Am J Gastroenterol* 2000; 95: 32–36.

Levine MS, Moolten DN, Herlinger H, *et al.* Esophageal intramural pseudodiverticulosis: a reevaluation. *Am J Roentgenol* 1986; 147: 1165–1170.

Monda L. Diagnosis and treatment of esophageal strictures. *Radio Technol.* 1999; 70: 361–372.

O'Connor JB, Richter JE: Esophageal strictures. In Castell DO, Richter JE (eds) *The Esophagus* 3rd edn, Philadelphia PA: Lippincott Williams & Wilkins; 1999.

Richter JE. Peptic strictures of the esophagus. *Gastroenterol Clin North Am* 1999; 28: 875–891.

Weinman D, Stewart M, Woodley DT, *et al*. Epidermolysis Bullosa Acquisita (EBA) and esophageal webs: a new association. *Am J Gastroenterol* 1991; 86: 1518–1522.

Chapter 7

Esophageal Cancer

David E. Loren and David A. Katzka

Esophageal carcinoma

Esophageal carcinoma remains a major cause of mortality despite an improved understanding of the etiologic and biologic features related to the disease. It is estimated that in 2002 there will be 13 100 new cases of esophageal cancer diagnosed in the US accompanied by 12 600 deaths from the disease. Generally, prognosis is poor as the overall 5-year survival is 14%, and for those with advanced disease, 5-year survival is below 2%.

Tumors of the esophagus can be subdivided into epithelial, non-epithelial, or metastatic types (Table 7.1), where adenocarcinoma and squamous cell carcinoma (SCCa) comprise the overwhelming majority of tumors. The discussion below will focus primarily on these two histologic subtypes, as they present the bulk of the management issues relating to esophageal neoplasms.

Epidemiology

Squamous cell carcinoma (Box 7.1)

Worldwide there is significant variation in the prevalence of esophageal cancers. In fact, more than half of the cases of esophageal SCCa occur in China, where there is observable clustering of cases, such that it is considered as endemic in particular regions. Other geographic areas of high prevalence of esophageal SCCa include Kazakhstan, Uzbekistan, Afghanistan, Iran, Singapore, por-

Table 7.1 Esophageal neoplasms

Tumor type	Clinical behavior
Epithelial – benign	
squamous cell papilloma	
Epithelial – malignant	
adenocarcinoma	aggressive
squamous cell carcinoma	aggressive
squamous cell carcinoma with spindle cell component	slow growing to aggressive
verrucous squamous cell carcinoma	slow growing to aggressive
adenocanthoma and adenosquamous carcinoma	aggressive
adenoid cystic carcinoma	aggressive
mucoepidermoid carcinoma	very aggressive
melanoma	very aggressive
carcinoid tumor	slow growing
small cell carcinoma	very aggressive
choriocarcinoma	aggressive
Non-epithelial – benign	
leiomyoma	
granular cell tumor	
fibrovascular polyp	
hemangioma/lymphangioma	
lipoma/fibroma	
Non-epithelial – malignant	
sarcoma	very aggressive
leiomyosarcoma	
Kaposi's sarcoma	
rhabdomyosarcoma	
neurogenic sarcoma	
lymphoma	varied depending on subtype
Hodgkin's disease	
non-Hodgkin's lymphoma	
Metastatic	
melanoma	
breast cancer	
other	

Box 7.1 Risk factors associated with esophageal squamous cell carcinoma

Environmental factors
alcohol use
cigarette smoking
mate-tea ingestion
betel-nut chewing
caustic ingestion
esophageal radiation exposure
diet high in saturated fat
diet low in vitamin C, folate, β-carotene,
  vitamin E

Demographic features
residing in an endemic region
male gender
African American race
low socioeconomic status

Associated medical conditions
presence of head/neck squamous cell cancer
Plummer–Vinson syndrome
achalasia
tylosis
celiac disease
human papilloma virus infection

tions of South Africa, and regions of the Indian subcontinent. Such geographical clustering suggests a significant contribution of environmental and genetic factors to the pathogenesis of the disease. Further support for an environmental influence on cancer development is the recognition of a correlation between regions of endemic esophageal cancer and the presence of gullet cancer in chickens. In high prevalence regions local animals would be exposed to similar environmental and perhaps dietary factors as humans, thus suggesting an etiologic link.

The prevalence of esophageal squamous cell carcinoma in the US has decreased slightly over recent decades. African Americans are more often affected than Caucasians in the US, and may carry a worse prognosis compared to whites. Men are affected more commonly than women in all racial subgroups in the US and around the world; however, the gender disparity is decreased in endemic areas. Lower socioeconomic status is an independent risk factor in the development of SCCa of the esophagus.

Alcohol and tobacco

A recent population-based case-control study in the US found that alcohol intake and cigarette smoking are associated with esophageal SCCa separate from racial and socioeconomic considerations. There appears to be a dose response regarding both alcohol consumption and the number of cigarettes smoked, further supporting the role of these factors in SCCa carcinogenesis. Moreover, quitting smoking can lower the risk of esophageal cancer, and prolonged abstinence from smoking enhances the risk reduction when compared to those who continue to smoke.

The chewing of betel nuts, a practice common in India and parts of Asia, is associated with a greater risk of esophageal SCCa. The effect of betel-nut chewing is independent of the contributions of tobacco and alcohol use.

Dietary factors

The role of diet in the incidence of esophageal SCCa has been implicated in a number of studies from around the world. Generally, a high intake of raw fruits and vegetables may be protective. High saturated-fat intake is associated with an increased incidence, whereas polyunsaturated fats have an inverse association with SCCa. When specific micronutrients are considered, there appears to be an inverse correlation with vitamin C, folate, β-carotene, and vitamin E which may be related to antioxidant properties of these foods. Intervention trials have failed to show a convincing benefit from vitamin supplementation in the reduction of esophageal cancer risk; however, lifetime supplementation may be required if a benefit is to be gained. Additionally, the ingestion of hot teas has been associated with the development of esophageal SSCa. In particular, the ingestion of mate tea, common in South America, demonstrates a significant dose-response correlation with SCCa risk. In addition to the tea itself, there appears to be an association with the temperature at the time of ingestion, with very hot tea having the highest risk.

Other risk factors

There are other, well-described risk factors that predispose individuals to esophageal SCCa. A diagnosis of squamous malignancy of the head or neck should warrant evaluation of the esophagus, as the concomitant development of esophageal cancer in this setting is well recognized. This phenomenon is a result of the common risk factors of smoking and tobacco for head and neck as well as esophageal squamous cancers. Tylosis, an autosomal dominant hereditary syndrome characterized by focal hyperkeratosis and pigmentation of the palms and soles, carries with it a 95% lifetime risk of developing esophageal squamous cell carcinoma. Plummer–Vinson syndrome composed of upper esophageal webs, iron deficiency, and koilonychia, is associated with carcinoma of the cervical esophagus. Reports of SCCa of the esophagus in individuals with celiac disease can be found in the literature; interestingly, celiac disease is also associated with Plummer–Vinson syndrome. Esophageal achalasia is associated with an increased risk of esophageal squamous neoplasia, in one study occurring in greater than 3% of those with achalasia, which corresponds to a 140-fold increase over the general population.

Caustic ingestion is a well-documented risk factor and imparts an estimated 1000-fold increase in cancer risk. In one case, a 10-month-old girl had ingested muriatic acid and died of esophageal cancer at age 10 years. Most often tumors are located in the mid-esophagus at the level of the tracheal bifurca-tion. Esophageal carcinoma has been found to arise within esophageal diverticula and duplication cysts, although because of the paucity of controlled data, it is not clear if there truly is an increased incidence in these settings. Esophageal exposure to radiation has been associated with esophageal SCCa and has been reported to occur in a multifocal pattern, suggesting a field effect from prior irradiation. Infectious etiologies have been suggested, in particular human papillomavirus, which may be associated with esophageal squamous cancer, and has been postulated as a contributor to the endemic incidence of disease in some areas.

Adenocarcinoma (Box 7.2)

Epidemiology

Similar to SCCa, esophageal adenocarcinoma is more common in males than females. However, in contrast to SCCa, adenocarcinoma occurs more commonly in Caucasians and higher socioeconomic strata. The incidence of the disease has been on the rise in the US as well as much of the world. Based upon Surveillance, Epidemiology, and End Results (SEER), database of the National Cancer Institute, there has been a continual rise over recent decades (see Figure 7.1). Increasing incidence has been observed in Australia and other western countries. Interestingly, the prevalence in Eastern Europe, which has the lowest incidence in Europe and one that is lower than the US and Australia, appears to have maintained a stable rate of occurrence of esophageal adenocarcinoma.

Barrett's metaplasia

Barrett's metaplasia, also known as Barrett's esophagus, is the presence of specialized intes-

Box 7.2 Risk factors associated with esophageal adenocarcinoma

Environmental factors
cigarette smoking
high-fat diet
diet low in vitamin C, folate, β-carotene, vitamin E

Demographic features
high socioeconomic status
Caucasian race
male gender

Associated medical conditions
Barrett's metaplasia
Zollinger–Ellison syndrome
scleroderma
prior esophageal dilations

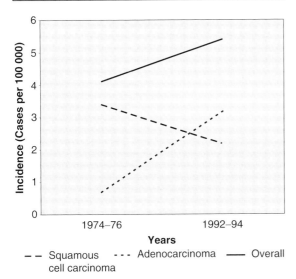

Figure 7.1 Changing incidence of esophageal carcinoma (adapted from Devesa SS, Blott WJ and Fraumeni JF Jr. Changing patterns in the incidence of esophageal and gastric carcinoma in the United States. *Cancer* 1998; 83: 2049–2053 copyright © 2003 American Cancer Society. Reprinted by permission of Wiley-Liss, Inc., a subsidiary of John Wiley & Sons, Inc.).

tinal metaplasia of the gastroesophageal junction, and is perhaps the most well-recognized risk for esophageal adenocarcinoma. While estimates vary, the rate of development of adenocarcinoma in patients with known Barrett's esophagus is generally believed to be approximately 0.5% per year. Barrett's metaplasia has been traditionally attributed to the reflux of gastric acid into the esophageal lumen resulting in mucosal damage and resultant changes in the epithelial lining. However, other factors such as the nature of refluxate (bile in addition to acid), duration of exposure of the esophageal mucosa to the refluxed material, and mucosal genetic factors all may be involved in this complex process. The resultant effect is a visible change of the normal whitish appearing squamous mucosa to a salmon-colored irregular mucosal appearance. Biopsy of the suspected area is required for diagnosis. Accordingly it is generally advocated that acid suppression with proton pump inhibitors be prescribed for those with Barrett's metaplasia, although it is not known if antisecretory treatment will affect the development of cancer.

Intuitively one would think that the larger the surface area of Barrett's mucosa, the greater the risk of cancer development, although this has not been convincingly demonstrated. Short segments of Barrett's mucosa, defined as less than 3 cm, carry a significant cancer risk, and are managed in the same manner as those with longer segments. The sequence of carcinogenesis is believed to be a progression from normal mucosa to metaplasia, dysplasia, and ultimately carcinoma. Accordingly, screening and surveillance programs are generally advocated to attempt to identify early stages in this succession, and thereby identify individuals who can undergo a curative procedure. There are data suggesting that endoscopic surveillance can identify less advanced lesions and improve survival better than using symptoms to prompt an evaluation.

Alcohol and tobacco

Tobacco appears to be a significant risk factor in the development of esophageal adenocarcinoma with studies demonstrating an increased risk with increased intensity and duration of tobacco use. Risk reduction following cessation is prolonged, requiring 30 years of abstinence to achieve a benefit. On the other hand, alcohol consumption does not appear to increase the risk of adenocarcinoma.

Dietary and other risk factors

The dietary considerations of esophageal adenocarcinoma are similar to those of squamous cell carcinoma, with the exception of the alcohol contribution; a diet that is high in overall fat intake has been associated with adenocarcinoma of the esophagus. It has been postulated that this effect may be related to an increase in gastroesophageal acid exposure related to high-fat diets rather than the dietary components themselves.

Other disease states that are associated with adenocarcinoma of the esophagus include the presence of scleroderma, Zollinger–Ellison syndrome, or having repeated esophageal dilations. The pathophysiology is though to be related to an increase in acid reflux in these settings, although disease-specific factors may confound the relationship.

Clinical presentation

Patients with esophageal cancer are usually detected because of the symptom of dysphagia, difficulty swallowing, which is the most common presenting symptom (Box 7.3). Initially, patients complain of difficulty swallowing solids and they may then progress to problems with liquid intake due to mechanical narrowing of the esophageal lumen. Occasionally, complete obstruction may occur prior to establishing the diagnosis. Odynophagia, painful swallowing, is also a common feature resulting from an ulcerated lesion. Chest pain, weight loss, anorexia, aspiration due to luminal obstruction, iron-defi-

Box 7.3 Clinical presentation of esophageal cancer

Dysphagia
Odynophagia
Chest pain
Anorexia
Weight Loss
Aspiration pneumonia
Anemia
Hemetemesis

ciency anemia, or hemetemesis may occur. The presence of constant chest pain in an individual with esophageal cancer is an ominous finding and suggests local invasion into the mediastinum. Patients with SCCa may present with hoarseness as a consequence of the proximal tumor location whether due to local factors, or involvement of the recurrent laryngeal nerve.

In endemic regions screening protocols may be used and thus the diagnosis can be made in asymptomatic patients. In China, a mesh-covered balloon is inserted through the mouth into the stomach, inflated, and pulled back, thus retrieving esophageal mucosal cells that undergo cytologic evaluation.

Diagnosis

Diagnostic evaluation

The first step in diagnosis is identification of the esophageal lesion. A careful history and physical examination in the patient complaining of dysphagia can lead the physician to an appropriate diagnostic test. For example, if, after a thorough history, one identifies progressive weight loss, esophageal cancer may be a consideration and endoscopic inspection would be indicated. Endoscopy allows for direct visualization of the lesion, evaluation of the extent of the mass, and provides a means of tissue acquisition. Additionally, other abnormalities such as the presence of Barrett's metaplasia can be identified, as well as alternative causes of symptoms such as benign strictures or esophagitis. Barium esophagram has been found to be an insensitive means of identification of neoplastic lesions, particularly early cancers, and performs unfavorably in the identification of Barrett's mucosa. Barium esophagram may be helpful in planning an endoscopic approach, as findings could direct one to schedule an endoscopic ultrasound at the same time as an upper endoscopy, and thus provide a more comprehensive and efficient staging of a lesion identified on the esophagram. Endoscopy with biopsy and cytologic brushings has been found to offer an accurate diagnosis in greater than 95% of cases and is the diagnostic study of choice. Chromoendoscopy, the application of surface stains to the mucosa at the time of endoscopy to highlight abnormal areas, may help identify subtle lesions. At the time of the evaluation the endoscopist will most commonly identify the lesion as either a mucosal irregularity, focal ulceration, exophytic mass, or stricture.

Clinical approach

The clinical approach to esophageal neoplasia varies with the tumor subtype, with consideration given to the histologic subtype, anatomic location of primary tumor, depth of invasion and locoregional metastasis, presence of distant metastases, clinical complaints, and performance status of the patient.

Anatomic considerations

When a patient is diagnosed with esophageal SCCa the traditional classification has been

according to its location in the proximal, middle, or distal third of the esophagus. More recently it has been advocated that tumor location be classified into the cervical esophagus, above the level of the tracheal bifurcation, and below the level of the tracheal bifurcation. Further description of the presence of invasion into the tracheobronchial tree of either the trachea or a mainstem bronchus, is important. The rationale behind this system is intrinsically related to the treatment strategies for management of esophageal SCCa.

Regarding esophageal adenocarcinoma, the most common anatomic presentation is at the gastroesophageal junction, and accordingly the initial approach is to distinguish between primary esophageal adenocarcinoma and adenocarcinoma of the gastric cardia, or of more distal gastric tumors that invade the distal esophagus. Generally, if more than 50% of a tumor is located in the esophagus then a primary esophageal tumor is diagnosed. The presence of Barrett's metaplasia adjacent to an adenocarcinoma of the distal esophagus strongly supports, but is not necessary for, the diagnosis of a primary esophageal lesion. The surgical approach to such a lesion will differ from that of one in which the majority of tumor is present in the stomach, as gastric cancer surgery is required. In addition, the anatomic evaluation should clearly identify the extent of Barrett's mucosa so that the entire segment can be removed should a surgery be performed.

Clinical staging

In addition to anatomic considerations, the approach to the evaluation of patients must offer an accurate assessment of both locoregional tumor and nodal staging and distant metastasis. The treatment strategy and prognosis should be evaluated by the TNM classification system for esophageal carcinoma of the American Joint Commission on Cancer Staging (Tables 7.2 and 7.3).

Endoscopic ultrasound

Endoscopic ultrasound (EUS) is the most accurate means of evaluating the extent of local tumor invasion and of regional lymphadenopathy. The proximity of the ultrasound probe to the esophageal mucosa offers a detailed characterization of the wall-layer pattern, and tumors can be seen to invade into the mucosa, submu-

Table 7.3 Stage grouping (from *American Joint Commission on Cancer Staging Manual* 5th edn, Philadelphia PA; Lippincott Williams & Wilkins: 1997)

Stage 0	Tis	N0	M0
Stage I	T1	N0	M0
Stage IIA	T2	N0	M0
	T3	N0	M0
Stage IIB	T1	N1	M0
	T2	N1	M0
Stage III	T3	N1	M0
	T4	N1	M0
Stage IV	Any T	Any N	M1
Stage IVA	Any T	Any N	M1a
Stage IVB	Any T	Any N	M1b

Table 7.2 TNM classification for esophageal cancer (from *American Joint Commission on Cancer Staging Manual* 5th edn, Philadelphia PA; Lippincott Williams & Wilkins: 1997)

Primary tumor (T)

TX   Primary tumor cannot be assessed
T0   No evidence of primary tumor
Tis   Carcinoma *in situ*
T1   Tumor invades lamina propria or submucosa
T2   Tumor invades muscularis propria
T3   Tumor invades adventitia
T4   Tumor invades adjacent structures

Regional lymph nodes (N)

NX   Regional lymph nodes cannot be assessed
N0   No regional lymph node metastasis
N1   Regional lymph node metastasis

Distant metastasis (M)

MX   Distant metastasis cannot be assessed
M0   No distant metastasis
M1   Distant metastasis
     Tumors of the lower thoracic esophagus
        M1a metastasis in celiac lymph nodes
        M1b other distant metastasis
     Tumors of the mid-thoracic esophagus
        M1a non-applicable
        M1b non-regional lymph nodes and/or other distant metastasis
     Tumors of the upper thoracic esophagus
        M1a metastasis in cervical nodes
        M1b other distant metastasis

cosa, muscularis propria, or serosa. Additionally, adjacent structures such as the trachea, aorta, and regional vasculature can be assessed for metastatic invasion. Lymphadenopathy of paraesophageal, paraaortic, paratracheal, and mediastinal locations can be seen, as well as identification of celiac axis lymphadenopathy. The identification of cancer metastasis to the celiac lymph nodes designates an individual unresectable for cure. Fine-needle aspiration of suspected pathologic nodes at the time of EUS is an important adjunct to endosonographic imaging, and can provide up to a 98% diagnostic accuracy in the setting of esophageal cancer. The primary limitations to the application of EUS for local staging include a stricture of the esophageal lumen that prevents passage of the echoendoscope. Luminal dilation to enable passage of the echoendoscope in this setting is controversial, as a high risk of perforation has been reported in some studies. Even so, individuals with luminal narrowing requiring esophageal dilation have a greater than 90% likelihood of having advanced-stage, inoperable disease. Another obstacle to complete EUS-directed staging is the absence of a biopsy track that is free of intervening tumor when biopsy of suspected lymphadenopathy is to be performed. Malignant cells may be picked up from the tumor rather than the lymph node of interest, thereby resulting in a falsely positive cytologic diagnosis from the aspirated material. In the situation when a biopsy is not performed, staging accuracy based on endosonographic features alone is approximately 90% for evaluation of the primary tumor, and 70% to 90% for lymphadenopathy.

Airway evaluation

Because of the increased risk of concurrent tumors of the head, neck, and lung in individuals with esophageal carcinoma, as well as concerns of involvement of the tracheo-bronchial tree from the primary tumor, consideration should be given to evaluation of these anatomic areas. This approach is most relevant for squamous esophageal neoplasms which share similar risk factors to cancers of the lung and airway, and arise in the more proximal esophagus, which has a close anatomic relationship to the adjacent airway, although bronchoscopy has been advocated for new cases of adenocarcinoma as well. Nasopharyngeal laryngoscopy provides direct visualization of the oropharynx and larynx, and bronchoscopy may identify bronchial impingement, concurrent mass, or fistula. Additionally, bronchial washings and cytologic brushings may identify malignancy that is not evident macroscopically. Up to one-third of patients will have macroscopic abnormalities at the time of airway evaluation.

Computed tomography

Computed tomography is a widely available imaging modality that offers excellent cross-sectional detail. The utility of CT in esophageal staging is most relevant for the identification of distant metastasis rather than primary tumor staging. Computed tomography compares poorly to EUS with fine-needle aspiration in determining the depth of tumor invasion and the presence of lymphadenopathy. Computed tomography assessment of lymph node invasion is based upon nodal size, and because nodal involvement by micrometastasis may not result in enlarged nodes, and because inflammatory changes in adjacent nodes can enlarge nodes without harboring malignancy, CT is inaccurate for this purpose. Computed tomography can evaluate for the common sites of metastasis, specifically the liver, lungs, adrenals, and kidneys, locations that are beyond the reach of EUS imaging.

Magnetic resonance imaging

Magnetic resonance imaging has little use in the staging of esophageal malignancy. It has not been shown to have superior test characteristics for local or distant metastasis when compared to EUS or CT. Thus it is used when other modalities cannot be performed.

Positron emission tomography

Positron emission tomography with fluorine-18 fluorodeoxyglucose (FDG-PET) is a newer technology that is not widely available, but performs well when used to identify metastatic implants. Fluorine-18 fluorodeoxyglucose is a radiopharmaceutical that can highlight areas of glucose metabolism, a process that is increased in rapidly dividing tumor cells. The ability of FDG-PET to detect locoregional lymphadenopathy is limited, particularly in the mid- and lower thoracic regions. Additionally, PET scan may be of prognostic importance in determining patient response to systemic chemotherapy. Thus FDG-PET scanning may become an increasingly relevant adjunct in the approach to the evaluation and management of the patient with esophageal cancer, although presently it has not been adapted as a standard study for patients with esophageal cancer.

Laparoscopic staging

Direct visualization and sampling of intra-abdominal viscera and nodes via laparoscopy has been advocated by some authorities, although it is not used in most centers as part of the routine staging of esophageal cancer.

Modes of spread

Tumors of the esophagus may spread by local invasion, lymphatic metastasis, or hematoge-nous spread to sites distant from the primary tumor. The most commonly encountered complication of local spread is obstruction of the esophageal lumen resulting in dysphagia, aspiration, and in severe cases complete esophageal obstruction. The manifestations of deep tumor invasion will depend upon the location of the invading mass. As discussed above, a proximal squamous cell carcinoma is more likely to cause a tracheo-esophageal fistula or damage the recurrent laryngeal nerve causing hoarseness, than would a more distal adenocarcinoma. Direct invasion into the aorta may result in catastrophic exsanguination, and local vertebral body invasion may cause pain or symptoms of spinal-cord compression. Extension into the peritoneal cavity may result in peritoneal carcinomatosis and associated bowel obstruction. Lymphatic spread occurs initially and rapidly to local nodes in the paraesophageal and paraaortic locations, as well as to paracardiac, left gastric, celiac, tracheobronchial, mediastinal, and supraclavicular sites. Even patients who have T1 tumors may already have lymph node involvement at the time of diagnosis. Hematogenous spread is most frequently to the liver, with pulmonary, adrenal, and renal metastasis being other common sites of disease.

Management

The optimal management of esophageal cancer is debated, and many of the studies are retrospective with limited follow-up; for a proposed algorithm for the evaluation and management, see Figure 7.2. What is clear is that early-stage disease limited to the esophageal wall has a much better prognosis than advanced-stage disease. Curative therapy is almost universally by means of surgical resection, thus patients who are inoperable are also, except for a few limited scenarios, incurable.

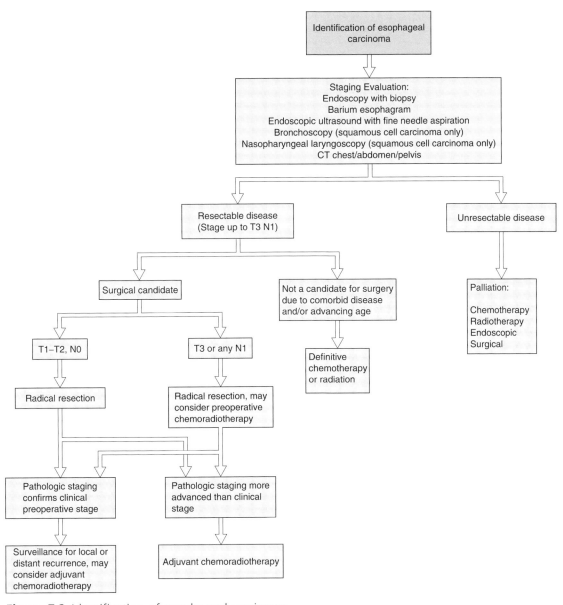

Figure 7.2 Identification of esophageal carcinoma.

Limitations to surgery are often not because of the tumor itself, but because of the comorbidities that occur in patients of advancing age and those accompanying major surgical procedures in these patients. Therefore, appraising a patient's performance status plays a central role in devising a treatment plan that will address tumor control and is tolerable to the patient.

Surgery

For cure of locoregional disease that is resectable, surgical removal offers the best chance of cure, yet the overall survival at 5 years is achieved in only 5% of patients who undergo surgery as single-modality therapy. Multimodality therapies have only resulted in a moderate improvement in survival. The morbidity attributed to esophagectomy has been decreasing over recent years but remains a significant consideration, especially for elderly patients who carry an operative risk of 10%.

The surgical procedure to be performed is determined by the anatomic location of the tumor as the primary factor. Approaches include transthoracic, transhiatal, and even transoral routes. Minimally invasive techniques using thoracoscopic and laparoscopic tools are gaining increasing attention. In every surgery performed with curative intent, the primary goal is complete resection of tumor and involved lymph nodes. This highlights the importance of a complete and accurate preoperative and intraoperative evaluation. In a patient who is a suitable candidate for esophagectomy based upon preoperative risk assessment, a surgery may not be attempted if there are involved lymph nodes beyond the surgical field, or if distant metastases are present. Thus anyone with disease up to clinical stage T3 N1 may be considered for surgical resection. However, a question that has not yet been adequately addressed is whether all resectable patients are potentially curable. This debate has become more complex as neoadjuvant therapies have become a mainstay of therapy in some centers. Nevertheless, the case remains that surgery offers the best hope for cure and prolonged survival, even for those with an expected poor 5-year survival.

Accompanying esophagectomy is the need for a replacement conduit to allow for food ingestion and accommodation. Most often this is through the mobilization of the stomach into the thorax, but colonic and jejunal interpositions have been performed. The functional outcome is usually acceptable, with patients generally able to eat and perform activities of daily living, although recovery to the preoperative state may be prolonged up to 2 years. Gastric mobilization is the most commonly performed procedure.

In situations where a cancer is found at an advanced stage of disease and complete resectability is not an option, surgical palliation may be considered. The application of endoscopic therapies, radiotherapy, and chemotherapy are reducing the number of palliative surgeries. However, in the case of a tracheoesophageal fistula, an esophageal bypass procedure may be necessary, although luminal esophageal stenting with a covered stent may offer adequate palliation.

Radiotherapy

The role of radiotherapy in the absence of concomitant chemotherapy is limited. The patient who is too ill to tolerate either surgery or chemotherapy may benefit from primary radiation therapy. The benefits are most often realized through palliation of dysphagia, and controlled prospective survival data are lacking. Radiation may be given as external beam radiation or as intraluminal brachytherapy. The latter approach may be used for lesions causing esophageal luminal obstruction.

Preoperative radiotherapy in an attempt to improve outcome does not appear to offer a survival benefit, with 2-year and 5-year survival being equivalent between those who received preoperative radiotherapy and those who did not. Regarding postoperative radiotherapy, a study from France of 221 patients identified a decreased local recurrence rate in those receiving adjuvant postoperative radiation. However, there was an increase in toxicities and a decrease in survival in the treatment group. Accordingly, adjuvant radiotherapy may be offered to those in whom surgery failed to achieve a complete resection in the hopes of decreasing the propensity of the residual tumor to recur.

Complications of radiotherapy include dysphagia and odynophagia due to esophagitis, esophageal ulceration, tracheo-esophageal fistula formation, and radiation-induced stricturing. Skin burns, myelitis, and pulmonary fibrosis have been reported to occur as a result of radiation therapy for esophageal cancers.

Chemotherapy

Chemotherapy plays a central role in the management of esophageal cancer, as one-third of patients will have metastatic disease at the time of diagnosis. Chemotherapy as primary therapy using cisplatin or 5-fluorouracil may result in response rates up to 40%, although a survival benefit has not been demonstrated. Generally, squamous cell carcinoma is thought to be more chemosensitive than adenocarcinoma, although this distinction has not been borne out in clinical studies.

Neoadjuvant chemotherapy has been used with the goal of eradicating micrometastasis in order to decrease the risk of recurrence. A large, multicenter, randomized trial failed to demonstrate a significant survival benefit to preoperative chemotherapy although there was a decreased risk of distant recurrence in the treatment group. Local recurrence was similar among treatment and control groups. Trials on postoperative chemotherapy have failed to demonstrate a survival benefit.

Combination chemoradiation

Chemotherapy combined with radiation therapy as definitive treatment has not been evaluated in controlled prospective trials when compared to surgery. For early-stage disease (T1 and T2 lesions) survival may be comparable to surgical resection, although surgery remains the standard of care. In a multicenter randomized trial of combination 5-fluorouracil, cisplatin, and radiotherapy versus radiotherapy alone, there was a 25% survival at 5 years in the combination therapy group, and no 5-year survivors in the radiation group. Thus, for patients who cannot tolerate a surgery, but may be candidates for chemoradiation, primary combination therapy may be a reasonable option.

The benefit to chemoradiation is believed to be in the neoadjuvant (preoperative) setting, although questions remain. All of the major trials have found a benefit to neoadjuvant combination therapy in some outcome parameters, although data are conflicting and not all outcomes have shown a benefit to treatment in all studies. Regimens typically are 5-fluorouracil and cisplatin based, combined with external beam radiation followed by surgery. If one combines the major trials, improved 3-year and 5-year survival as well as decreased locoregional recurrence have been demonstrated. Benefits from combination preoperative therapy have been observed for both adenocarcinoma and squamous cell carcinoma.

Palliation (Box 7.4)

Unfortunately, more than one-half of patients present with unresectable disease and must be considered for palliative approaches. Surgical palliation with esophagectomy or bypass procedures have resulted in high complication rates and are generally reserved for those who have failed other therapies. A bypass may be warranted in the case of tracheo-esophageal fistulas or when the expected survival may be longer than 6 months. Radiotherapy, often administered over 3 weeks, can provide palliation of dysphagia; however, acute esophagitis as well as strictures over the longer term may result. Endoscopic treatments are becoming increasingly used and include luminal stenting with expandable metal stents, dilation therapy, laser fulguration of tumor, local electrocautery,

---

Box 7.4 Palliation of esophageal cancer

Surgical palliation
esophagectomy
esophageal bypass surgery

Endoscopic palliation
tumor tissue destruction
   laser
   argon plasma coagulation
   electrocautery
   photodynamic therapy
   brachytherapy
esophageal stenting
esophageal dilation

Other
radiotherapy
chemotherapy

---

photodynamic therapy, and intraluminal brachytherapy. Photodynamic therapy in particular is often used for patients who are non-operative candidates and have been diagnosed with superficial lesions of high-grade dysplasia or carcinoma-in-situ arising in the setting of Barrett's metaplasia. Palliative systemic chemotherapy may be administered to patients with systemic metastasis and an adequate performance status.

Other esophageal tumors

There is a wide spectrum of lesions that may be encountered in the esophagus. These include other primary epithelial lesions as well as non-epithelial lesions and metastatic tumors. The tumor types vary in their clinical behavior and malignant potential and are listed in Table 7.1. Similar to SCCa and adenocarcinoma, the approach to the management of these tumors depends upon the histology and location of the lesion.

A common presentation of esophageal lesions that warrants further consideration is the endoscopic finding of a subepithelial lesion of the esophagus. These are often discovered as an incidental finding when an endoscopy is performed for unrelated symptoms, or when an abnormality is seen on another imaging study such as a barium esophagram or CT scan. A subepithelial lesion is described by a visible, distinct impression that is made upon the esophageal lumen, yet the overlying mucosa appears normal and is intact. The differential diagnosis of subepithelial lesions includes abnormalities of the esophageal wall such as a lipomas, stromal cell tumors, Schwannomas, granular cell tumors, esophageal duplication cysts and lymphatic cysts, as well as lesions outside the mural esophagus. Extrinsic compression from extramural lesions includes benign processes such as vascular structures, benign lymphadenopathy, and bronchial cysts. Malignant subepithelial lesions may be the result of primary cancers of adjacent organs, metastatic implants, or malignant lymphadenopathy. The evaluation of subepithelial tumors generally includes an EUS along with cross-sectional imaging. Endoscopic ultrasound can offer excellent local detail including delineation of mural from extramural lesions, and it can identify features characteristic of lipomas, leiomyomas, and cancers, whereas cross-sectional studies allow for identification of associated regional and distant abnormalities (e.g. aortic aneurysm, metastases, diffuse lymphadenopathy). Endoscopic ultrasound-directed fine-needle aspiration adds additional information by providing tissue for histologic diagnosis; however, because of limitations of cytologic analysis, fine-needle aspiration is not helpful in all cases. For lesions arising from the esophageal wall, it has been suggested that the EUS findings of echogenic foci, an irregular border, cystic degeneration, and large size correlate with malignancy and warrant further management. Additionally, molecular markers such as c-KIT, a marker found almost universally in gastrointestinal stromal tumors, will continue to emerge as important diagnostic tools. Surgical resection of lesions may be warranted if there is concern of cancer due to tumor features such as size or echofeatures, or if malignant cells are diagnosed on fine-needle aspiration or other means of tissue acquisition, and no other contraindication to surgery exists. Prognosis depends on the histology of the lesion and presence of metastatic lesions.

Further reading

Blazeby JM, Farndon JR, Donovan J, Alderson D. A prospective longitudinal study examining the quality of life of patients with esophageal carcinoma. *Cancer* 2000; 88: 1781–1787.

Bollschweiler E, Wolfgarten E, Gutschow C, Holscher AH. Demographic variations in the rising incidence of esophageal adencocarcinoma in white males. *Cancer* 2001; 92: 549–555.

Botet JF, Lightdale CJ, Zauber AG, Gardes H, Urmacher C, Brennan MF. Preoperative staging of esophageal cancer: comparison of endoscopic US and dynamic CT. *Radiology* 1991; 181: 419–425.

Castellsague X, Munoz N, De Stefani E, Victora CG, Castelletto R, Rolon PA. Influence of mate drinking, hot beverages and diet on esophageal cancer risk in South America. *Int J Cancer* 2000; 88: 658–664.

Cooper JS, Guo MD, Herskovic A, *et al.* Chemoradiotherapy of locally advanced esophageal cancer: long-term follow-up of a prospective randomized trial (RTOG 85-01). Radiation Therapy Oncology Group. *JAMA* 1999; 281: 1623–1627.

Corley DA, Levin TR, Habel LA, Weiss NS, Buffler PA. Surveillance and survival in Barrett's adenocarcinomas: a population-based study. *Gastroenterology* 2002; 122: 633–640.

Eloubeidi MA, Wallace MB, Reed CE, *et al.* The utility of EUS and EUS-guided fine needle aspiration in detecting celiac lymph node metastasis in patients with esophageal cancer: a single-center experience. *Gastrointest Endosc* 2001; 54: 714–719.

Kato H, Kuwano H, Nakajima M, *et al.* Comparison between positron emission tomography and computed tomography in the use of the assessment of esophageal carcinoma. *Cancer* 2002; 94: 921–928.

Kelsen DP, Ginsberg R, Pajak TF, *et al.* Chemotherapy followed by surgery compared with surgery alone for localized esophageal cancer. *N Engl J Med* 1998; 339: 1979–1984.

Mayne ST, Risch HA, Dubrow R, *et al.* Nutrient intake and risk of subtypes of esophageal and gastric cancer. *Cancer Epidemiol Biomarkers Prev* 2001; 10: 1055–1062.

Spechler SJ. Clinical practice, Barrett's Esophagus, *N Engl J Med* 2002; 346: 836–842.

Stein HJ, Brucher BL, Sendler A, Slewert JR. Esophageal cancer: patient evaluation and pretreatment staging. *Surg Oncol* 2001; 10: 03–111.

Wajed SA, Peters JH, Laparoscopic and endoscopic surgery in esophageal malignancy. *Surg Oncol Clin N Am* 2001; 10: 493–510, vii.

Walsh TN, Noonan N, Hollywood D, Kelly A, Keeling N, Hennessy TP. A comparison of multimodal therapy and surgery for esophageal adenocarcinoma. *N Engl J Med* 1996; 335: 462–467.

Wong R, Malthaner R. Esophageal cancer: a systematic review. *Curr Probl Cancer* 2000; 24: 297–373.

Chapter 8

Helicobacter pylori Gastritis and Other Gastric Infections

David C. Metz and Yu-Xiao Yang

CHAPTER OUTLINE

Introduction

The role of *Helicobacter pylori* in the causation of peptic ulcers is now generally accepted although this was controversial when Drs. Marshall and Warren first discovered it in 1983. The epidemiology of *H. pylori* suggests that it is acquired in early childhood and that transmission is via the fecal–oral route, especially in areas with poor sanitation. Consequently, the organism is much more common in developing countries than in the developed world (Figure 8.1). In developing countries, people acquire the infection at an early age, and by young adulthood as many as 90% of the population might have *H. pylori* gastritis. In developed western countries such as the US, the prevalence of *H. pylori* gastritis is much lower. Under these conditions, the rate of acquisition is much slower (less than 1% per annum), and the older a person is, the more likely they are to be infected with the organism. However, this phenomenon is likely to reflect improved living conditions in the US over the past 50 years rather than being truly age related, as most of these elderly patients were probably infected when they were young.

Published data from a few years ago established that approximately 70% of all gastric ulcers were due to infection with *H. pylori*. The corresponding figure for duodenal ulcers was over 90%. However, combining data from six large, well-controlled trials in the US, a recent study evaluated more than 2000 patients with endoscopically diagnosed, non-NSAID, duodenal ulcers and found that the *H. pylori* infection rate was only 73%. Another population-based study in Rochester, NY found that only 42% to 61% of patients with peptic ulcer disease were infected with *H. pylori*. Age-specific analysis showed that younger patients with ulcers were more likely to be infected and that the incidence of NSAID-related ulcers increased with age (see Chapter 9). The preva-

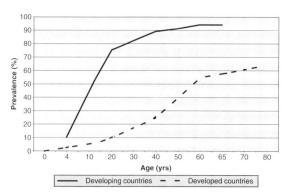

Figure 8.1 *Helicobacter pylori* prevalence in developed and developing countries (adapted with permission from Logan RP, Walker MM. ABC of the upper gastrointestinal tract: epidemiology and diagnosis of *Helicobacter pylori* infection. *BMJ* 2001; 323: 920–922).

lence of *H. pylori* infection was much higher in non-Caucasians than in Caucasians. Furthermore, 42% of the patients with peptic ulcers in the study were both *H. pylori* negative and NSAID negative. It is unclear whether these data represent under-reporting of NSAID use by the patients or whether they implicate the presence of additional unknown important causative factors for peptic ulcer disease. Nevertheless, the lower prevalence of *H. pylori* infection provides evidence against the use of empirical antibiotic therapy for uncharacterized peptic ulcers.

Pathogenesis

Helicobacter pylori is a spiral, gram-negative bacterium that colonizes the human gastric mucosa. The organism is found in the mucus layer and adheres to the surface mucous epithelium of the stomach but generally does not penetrate the gastric mucosa directly. However, there is a secondary inflammatory response in the mucosa leading to chronic active gastritis. In order for *H. pylori* to colonize the duodenum, gastric metaplasia is

required. The presence of gastric surface mucous cells in this location permits adherence of the organism and appears to be important in the development of *H. pylori*-associated duodenal ulcers. A humoral immune response with circulating antibodies also occurs. One of *H. pylori*'s more important enzyme products is urease, which may have a protective function by providing an alkaline micro-environment for the organism within the gastric lumen. Whether *H. pylori* gastritis itself causes symptomatic disease or not is yet to be resolved, although the prevailing theory at present is that *H. pylori* itself is asymptomatic. Koch's postulate is fulfilled with regards to the gastritis itself, in that infection leads to histologic gastritis, which resolves with successful antibiotic therapy. *H. pylori* infection is associated with a number of apparently unrelated disease states (Box 8.1).

There is a very strong association between the presence of *H. pylori* gastritis and the development of both duodenal and gastric ulcers. The strongest evidence in favor of these associations comes from therapeutic trials using antibiotics to cure *H. pylori* gastritis in patients with active peptic ulcer disease. Patients given antibiotics in addition to standard anti-secretory therapy were noted to heal peptic ulcers more rapidly, as well as to have a much lower incidence of recurrence after healing as compared with those who received standard anti-secretory therapy alone. Among those who heal their duodenal ulcers after failed *H. pylori* eradication treatment, persistent infection with *H. pylori* is

Box 8.1 Disease states associated with *Helicobacter pylori* infection

Gastritis
Duodenal ulcers
Gastric ulcers
Gastric cancer
Maltoma
Others are postulated but not proven

associated with a much higher ulcer recurrence rate. An important issue that remains to be clarified in patients with *H. pylori* gastritis is an understanding of who among the infected population is at risk for the subsequent development of peptic ulcer disease. Patients in the developing world tend to have a high prevalence of *H. pylori* gastritis but a low incidence of peptic ulceration. It has been estimated that approximately one in six infected persons in the US will ultimately develop a peptic ulcer. *Helicobacter pylori* may predispose to peptic ulcer formation in a variety of ways. Early theories implicated bacterial urease as playing a directly toxic role. However, urease is not currently felt to be directly causative in either the underlying gastritis or in the development of peptic ulceration, although it likely is important in facilitating colonization of the stomach. The variable outcomes of *H. pylori* infection appear to be associated with the location of the gastritis and its effects on gastric physiology. During the first few months of *H. pylori* infection, acute gastritis results in a marked decrease in gastric-acid secretion. Following the acute hypochlorhydria, chronic *H. pylori* infection is linked with three potential patterns of acid secretion:

- hyposecretion associated with chronic atrophic pangastritis
- hypersecretion from antral predominant infection
- normosecretion in most asymptomatic carriers (Figure 8.2).

The predominant location of *H. pylori* gastritis determines its influence on the risks of developing peptic ulcers, gastric cancer, and GERD (Figure 8.3). The World Health Organization and International Agency for Research on Cancer consensus group stated in 1994 that there was sufficient epidemiologic and histologic evidence to classify *H. pylori* as a definite carcinogen for gastric cancer. A recent large study from Japan found that gastric cancer develops in persons infected with *H. pylori* but not in uninfected persons. Most other recent studies also have found *H. pylori* to be positively associated with gastric cancer. The consequence of *H. pylori* eradication also differs depending on the pattern of *H. pylori* infection before treatment.

The precise reason for the varied acid profile in chronic *H. pylori* infection is unclear, but it may be related to organism virulence factors, differences in host responses, environmental cofactors, proton pump inhibitor therapy, and age at onset of infection (Table 8.1).

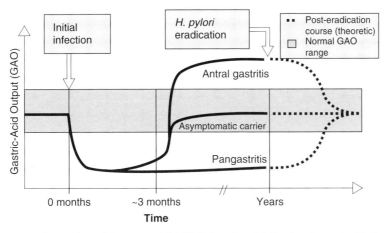

Figure 8.2 Patterns of gastric-acid output (GAO) following *Helicobacter pylori* infection.

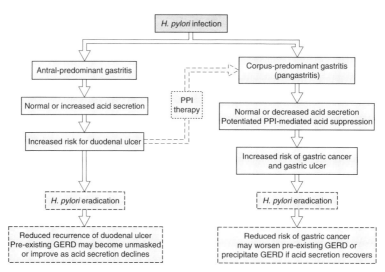

Figure 8.3 Consequences of antral-predominant and corpus-predominant *Helicobacter pylori* gastritis (shaded areas are theoretic, i.e. not proven). PPI proton pump inhibitor.

Helicobacter pylori produces a variety of cellular mediators and enzymes that cause ulceration directly or predispose to ulcer formation by promoting a mucosal inflammatory response in the human host. Using molecular biologic techniques, investigators have identified bacterial gene products (including Cag A, Vac A, and, more recently, Cag B, C, and E) that appear to be important with regard to the development of clinically significant disease in infected persons. Vac A is produced by all *H. pylori* strains and encodes a cytotoxin. It has at

Table 8.1 Potential factors affecting gastric-acid output following *Helicobacter pylori* infection

Potential factors		Effect
Organism	Virulence factor Cag A	more severe corpus gastritis
		more atrophic gastritis
		more gastric cancer
		more peptic ulcers
	Other virulence factors (e.g. Vac A s1, IceA1)	more peptic ulcers
Host	Blood type (type O)	more pangastritis
		more gastric ulcers
	Blood type (type A)	more gastric cancer
	Interleukin-1 gene cluster polymorphisms	more gastric cancer
	Class II antigen subtypes (DQ-B-type DQ5)	more atrophic gastritis
Environmental	Proton pump inhibitor therapy	more pangastritis
	Antioxidants (e.g. vitamins C and B)	protective against atrophy
	Excessive sodium intake	more atrophic gastritis
	Others (smoking)	more atrophic gastritis

least four Vac A signal sequence types (s1a, s1b, s1c, and s2) and three middle region types (m1, m2 a and m2 b). The various subtypes of Vac A confer different levels of cytotoxicity. Cag A is not present in all strains of *H. pylori*. It marks the presence of a pathogenicity island in the bacterial genome, whose gene products can result in more severe gastritis through enhanced cytokine induction. The Cag A, Cag E and Vac A s1 genotypes are more prevalent among patients with peptic ulcer disease, again suggesting that these may be important virulence factors.

Helicobacter pylori infection has significant influences on gastric physiology. Infected individuals have increased basal serum gastrin levels. Patients with *H. pylori* gastritis have increased serum gastrin levels possibly due to a local somatostatin deficiency from gastritis-induced inhibition of gastric mucosal D cells in the antrum. The hypergastrinemia in turn may lead to relative gastric-acid hypersecretion in some patients, a common finding in patients with idiopathic duodenal ulcer disease. Studies have shown that cure of the gastritis leads to normalization of the hypergastrinemia, suggesting a causative role for the infection in the hypergastrinemia itself. Moreover, there are now good data to suggest that reversibility also occurs with regard to the underlying relative gastric-acid hypersecretion. It is likely, there-fore, that *H. pylori* gastritis causes duodenal ulceration via a combination of two mechanisms: a reduction in cytoprotection as well as a relative increase in gastric-acid secretion. In pangastritis, hypergastrinemia is from hyposecretion, but enough acid is secreted to permit peptic ulceration because mucosal defense is impaired by the inflammatory response. Most patients with *H. pylori* infection are normo-secretors and therefore do not develop peptic ulcers.

Clinical presentation

The gastritis itself is felt to be asymptomatic in most patients. However, patients can certainly present with peptic-ulcer-related symptoms or complications (see Chapter 9). *Helicobacter pylori* gastritis has also been associated with the development of gastric cancer and gastric lymphomas, including lymphomas of mucosal-associated lymphoid tissue (maltomas) (Table 8.2). However, its association with non-ulcer dyspepsia, an extremely common disorder that affects as much as 30% of the general population in the US, is not yet clear. A recent study suggested that eradicating *H. pylori* infection does not impact on non-ulcer dyspepsia symptoms.

Table 8.2 *Helicobacter pylori* infection and gastric malignancies	
Gastric Cancer	90% of distal gastric cancers are associated with *Helicobacter pylori* infection.
	Helicobacter pylori eradication may prevent progression of early gastric cancer.
	Test-and-treat strategy to prevent gastric cancer may be cost effective.
	Gastric cancer is more likely in Cag A-positive *Helicobacter pylori* infection.
Maltoma	Maltoma can rarely arise in *Helicobacter pylori*-induced chronic gastritis.
	More than 90% of gastric maltomas are associated with *Helicobacter pylori* infection.
	Maltoma often regresses with antibiotics.

Table 8.3 Invasive and non-invasive diagnostic methods for *Helicobacter pylori* infection

Modality		Sensitivity (%)	Specifity (%)
Invasive methods (endoscopic antral biopsy)			
Rapid urease tests of biopsy specimen (CLO test)		89.6	100
Culture of biopsy specimen		variable	100
Histological identification		93.1	99
Non-invasive methods			
Serological testing*	Quantitative enzyme-linked immunosorbent assay (ELISA)	97	94
	Qualitative rapid office-based tests	76–90	90–98
Breath tests	Carbon-13 (non-radioactive)	90.2	95.8
	Carbon-14 (radioactive)	90.2	95.8
Antigen-based assay	Stool antigen test	94	91

* not useful for active infection or documentation of eradication; acceptable accuracy in high-prevalence areas

Diagnosis

The diagnosis of *Helicobacter pylori* gastritis may be made using invasive or non-invasive methods (Table 8.3). The non-invasive methods detect the organism indirectly by identifying a humoral immune response to the infection (antibody testing) or by detecting bacterial urease, an enzyme product unique to *H. pylori* organisms (urea breath tests). *Helicobacter pylori* antigens can also be identified in stool specimens. The invasive diagnostic methods are either indirect (rapid urease tests of biopsy specimens) or direct (bacterial culture or histologic identification with appropriate stains). The gold standard for the diagnosis of *H. pylori* gastritis is identification of *H. pylori* organisms with endoscopic biopsy (at least two antral specimens taken 3 to 5 cm from the pylorus). Although routine histology with hematoxylin and eosin is the standard method for diagnosing inflammation (i.e. the gastritis itself), it may be difficult to identify *H. pylori* organisms accurately with this stain.

Special stains such as the Giemsa, Warthin Starry, or Genta, provide better sensitivity and specificity for diagnosing *H. pylori* gastritis. Studies have indicated accuracy as high as 98% for histology using these staining techniques. Even with special stains, however, a potential disadvantage of histology for the diagnosis of *H. pylori* gastritis in clinical practice is the possibility of inter- and intra-observer variability in detecting organisms. The most specific method of diagnosing *H. pylori* gastritis is culture of antral biopsy specimens. This method, however, has not become routine in most clinical settings because *H. pylori* is a fastidious organism that is difficult to culture. In specialized centers cultures are becoming increasingly useful for detecting antibiotic resistance in specific individuals who fail attempted antibiotic cure of their infections. Rapid urease testing (e.g. *Campylobacter*-like organism (CLO) testing) is a highly effective method for the detection of *H. pylori* gastritis that is independent of inter- or intra-observer variability. The CLO test appears to be very accurate, with a sensitivity and specificity of more than 90%. Newer diagnostic techniques have focused on performing polymerase chain reactions on biopsy or other samples (stool or gastric juice). *In situ* hybridization techniques have also been developed. It is unlikely, however, that these

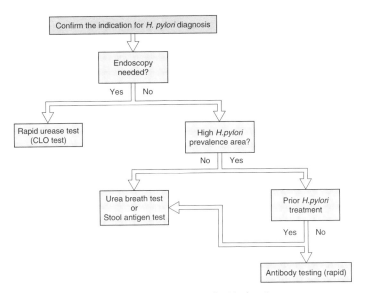

Figure 8.4 Diagnostic algorithm for *Helicobacter pylori* infection.

techniques will add significantly to currently available tests, except in specialized research situations in which *H. pylori* subtyping is required. Many investigators favor biopsies for both histology and CLO testing during endoscopy although this approach is expensive and CLO testing alone is quite accurate. A false-negative CLO test can always be readily excluded by antibody testing. In patients with bleeding peptic ulcers, rapid urease testing has been shown to lack sensitivity. Concomitant proton pump inhibitor therapy decreases the yield of the CLO test. This problem can be mitigated to some extent by biopsying the fundus as well as the antrum of the stomach. True absence of *H. pylori* gastritis in patients with documented ulcer disease should alert the physician to the possibility of other etiologies such as NSAID-induced ulcers and Zollinger–Ellison syndrome (Chapter 9).

Antral biopsies should always be performed if an ulcer is identified during upper endoscopy. However, patients should not undergo endoscopy purely for the diagnosis of *H. pylori* gastritis if they have, for example, a prior history of peptic ulceration (Figure 8.4). Non-invasive testing should be the primary approach in this situation. Serologic testing is simple to perform and widely available. There does not appear to be any advantage to performing immunoglobulin-A antibody testing in addition to immunoglobulin-G antibody testing. Serologic tests are highly sensitive and specific but cannot distinguish readily between the serologic scar of previous *H. pylori* exposure and active infection. Nevertheless, most patients with *H. pylori* gastritis develop their infections early on in life, and these infections persist. Spontaneous clearance of the organism is unusual, and monotherapy antibiotic regimens that may have been given to patients with urinary tract infections or other minor infections generally fail to cure *H. pylori* gastritis. Therefore, it is reasonable to assume that a positive antibody test implies active gastritis, unless the patient has received specific anti-*H. pylori* therapy previously. Both qualitative and quantitative serologic tests are available. The qualitative tests are most useful as rapid office-based tests. Laboratory-based serology tests are able to quantify the amount of antibody present by using an enzyme-linked immunosorbent assay (ELISA). The advantage of serial ELISA testing is that, with prolonged follow-up after therapy, patients can be classified as cured if their ELISA levels decrease significantly, but this is a cumbersome approach, and is no longer recommended. Serologic testing should not be used in low prevalence areas because the high likelihood of a false-positive result outweighs its potential benefits (i.e. lower cost, ease of use) compared with breath testing.

Breath testing is especially useful for documenting cure of *H. pylori* gastritis after antibiotic therapy. There are two breath tests. The carbon-13 urea breath test has the advantage of being non-radioactive, but it is more expensive and somewhat cumbersome to perform. In addition, carbon-13 breath testing still requires a mass spectroscopy unit which is not generally available. Therefore, most patients undergoing this form of breath testing will have their test performed at a remote site. The carbon-14 urea breath test is a similar test. It has the advantage of not requiring a pre-dose meal, and the test itself can be readily performed using a standard scintillation counter available at most major medical centers. The disadvantage of this method is the small dose of radiation exposure. The test currently approved in the US is a 1-μCi test that provides radiation equivalent to one thirtieth of a chest X-ray per test. In practice, the urea breath test is now regarded as the diagnostic method of choice in patients who do not need endoscopy.

Stool antigen testing has recently emerged as an accurate, rapid, non-invasive modality of *H. pylori* detection. A recent study reported a sensitivity of 94% and a specificity of 90% for the primary diagnosis of *H. pylori* infection in symptomatic patients. When used for assessing eradication of *H. pylori* infection, the stool antigen test was found by the same authors to have a sensitivity of 95.6% and a specificity of 94.7%. However, results from other studies that assessed the accuracy of the stool antigen test for docu-

menting eradication after *H. pylori* treatment have not been as encouraging.

An important point regarding the diagnosis of *H. pylori* gastritis using both invasive and non-invasive testing methods is that testing needs to be done in the appropriate clinical setting. For determination of cure status, testing should not be performed any sooner than 4 weeks after completion of the antibiotic regimen. This is necessary to distinguish between antibiotic-induced suppression of *H. pylori* gastritis and true cure. A second important point is that all methods of detecting *H. pylori* gastritis (except for antibody tests) are dependent on the presence of medications that may suppress the organism, thus giving the false impression of a cure. About 33% of *H. pylori*-positive patients develop false-negative urea breath tests while taking proton pump inhibitors. Most patients infected with *H. pylori* will revert to positive urea breath test results by 1 week after the discontinuation of proton pump inhibitor therapy. Based on these results, patients should stop taking proton pump inhibitors for 2 weeks before undergoing urea breath testing for *H. pylori* infection.

As a general guideline, one should not test for *H. pylori* infection if there is no intention of treating it if the test is positive (Box 8.2). Gastroesophageal reflux disease is not an indication for *H. pylori* testing. In fact, *H. pylori* infection may be protective against GERD. No association between functional dyspepsia and

Box 8.2 General guidelines for testing for *Helicobacter pylori* infection

Do not test if not intending to treat if positive
Do not test GERD patients
Testing for functional dyspepsia not warranted
Test (and treat) all documented ulcer patients
Test (and treat) non-specific dyspepsia in young patients
Test (and treat) maltoma patients
Testing (and treating) to reduce gastric cancer not standard of care

H. pylori infection has been demonstrated. Therefore, testing for *H. pylori* infection in patients with functional dyspepsia is not warranted. In young patients without warning signs (e.g. weight loss, anemia), a test- and-treat strategy is appropriate. *Helicobacter pylori* infection should be sought and eradicated if present in patients with established peptic ulcer disease or maltoma because of the well-known causal association between *H. pylori* infection and these two conditions. Finally, although *H. pylori* infection has been linked with the development of gastric cancer, testing for and treating *H. pylori* infection in an effort to reduce gastric cancer is currently not the standard of care. The 1994 National Institutes of Health consensus conference on *H. pylori* and peptic ulcer disease came out strongly in favor of the use of antibiotic therapy in patients who have *H. pylori*-associated ulcers. This consensus conference also recommended that patients should be treated for *H. pylori* only following documentation of the infection and stopped short of recommending therapy for patients with *H. pylori* gastritis in the absence of ulcer disease, whether or not they had symptoms (Table 8.4).

Treatment

Successful administration of antibiotics in combination with histamine H_2-receptor antagonists or proton pump inhibitors accelerates healing of *Helicobacter pylori*-associated duodenal and gastric ulcers. A more important benefit of successful antibiotic therapy, however, is that duodenal and gastric ulcer relapse is greatly diminished or virtually eliminated after cure of the gastritis in such patients. There are also data suggesting that antibiotic therapy may decrease the likelihood of ulcer complications. Thus, antibiotic treatment for the underlying gastric infection results in a cure of the peptic ulcer disease in patients with *H. pylori*-associated ulceration. In addition, maltomas often respond to *H. pylori* eradication.

The optimal therapeutic regimen for curing *H. pylori* gastritis is not yet established (Table 8.5). Triple therapy with metronidazole, a bismuth compound, and tetracycline has now been supplanted by proton pump inhibitor-based triple therapy consisting of a proton pump inhibitor and two antibiotics (either metronidazole, clarithromycin, or ampicillin) The cure rate after completion of at least 10 full days of proton pump inhibitor-based triple therapy is well over 90%, and the therapy is generally well tolerated. However, these results may decrease as clarithromycin resistance increases. First-line therapy is proton pump inhibitor-based clarithromycin triple therapy as long as the patient has not received clarithromycin before. Because of

Table 8.4 The pros and cons of *Helicobacter pylori* eradication	
Pros	Cons
Decreased peptic ulcer disease relapse.	Possible delayed NSAID ulcer healing (theoretic concern).
Decreased likelihood of ulcer complications.	Possible increase in GERD and GERD-associated complications, e.g. Barrett's esophagus and esophageal adenocarcinoma (theoretic concern).
Possibly decreased risk of gastric cancer (even with early disease).	
Regression of maltoma.	Possible increased development of antibiotic resistance.

Table 8.5 *Helicobacter pylori* eradication regimens

Regimen (%)	Duration of treatment (days)	Eradication (%)	Non-compliance adjusted eradication (%)
PCA*	14	89	82
PCM**	10–14	91	84
PMA	10–14	84	76
PBMT#	10–14	96	85
BMT	14	90	80
BMA	14	70	62
PC##	14	72	65
PA##	14	63	58

P: proton pump inhibitor; B: bismuth; M: metronidazole; T: tetracycline; C: clarithromycin; A: amoxicillin.
* recommended first-line regimen.
** alternative first-line regimen if + penicillin allergy.
\# salvage regimen.
\#\# dual therapy is not recommended (potential for inducing antibiotic resistance).

the relatively high rate of metronidazole resistance, amoxicillin should be used unless there is penicillin allergy.

Other useful regimens include another combination agent, ranitidine bismuth citrate (no longer available in the US), with various antibiotics as triple (e.g. with clarithromycin or metronidazole) or quadruple therapy (e.g. with clarithromycin or metronidazole plus amoxicillin). The ultimate aim is to identify an antibiotic regimen that is virtually 100% effective with good tolerability. Following therapy to cure patients of *H. pylori* gastritis one can expect recurrence rates for peptic ulcer disease to drop from 80% to virtually 0% at 1 year.

Role of confirmatory testing after eradication therapy

Performing confirmatory testing to document *Helicobacter pylori* eradication in all patients is clearly not cost effective. Patients who are not cured of *H. pylori* infection, however, are still at risk for ulcer recurrence despite initial healing of their ulcers. It is especially important to document cure in patients who presented with ulcer complications such as bleeding, before stopping maintenance anti-secretory therapy, while patients with a history of uncomplicated ulcer disease should have follow-up testing only if symptoms recur (Figure 8.5). There is little justification for performing an upper endoscopy for the sole purpose of diagnosing *H. pylori* gastritis in patients who are symptom free. Serial antibody levels are useful only if pretreatment serum is stored and then paired with post-treatment serum a number of months later. The definition of a diagnostic decrease in antibody levels is as yet unclear, and the appropriate timing for post-treatment testing has not been accurately defined. This cumbersome approach is not recommended. Urea breath testing is the non-invasive method of choice for documenting cure of *H. pylori* gastritis after antibiotic therapy. Recent studies have suggested that *H. pylori* stool antigen testing may be as accurate. The main reasons for failure of *H. pylori* eradication therapy are non-compliance and antimicrobial resistance. Therefore, patients with confirmed persistent infection should be

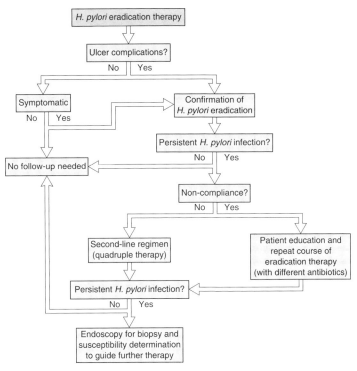

Figure 8.5 Algorithm for follow-up testing after *Helicobacter pylori* eradication therapy.

assessed for treatment non-compliance. In addition, alternative regimens should be considered. Quadruple therapy for 14 days is a reasonable second-line treatment that is effective in most patients who failed regimens containing clarithromycin and in some who failed a metronidazole-containing regimen. For those patients who do not respond to a second course of eradication therapy, endoscopy with biopsy and culture for the determination of *H. pylori* susceptibility is required. Further therapy will be guided by the culture and susceptibility results.

Other gastric infections and gastritis

Gastric infections other than *Helicobacter pylori* rarely occur in healthy people. However, they

can develop in patients with compromised immunity or elevated gastric pH (Table 8.6). It is generally believed that low pH in the stomach acts as a barrier for infection. Patients with metaplastic atrophic gastritis, post–gastrectomy patients, the elderly, alcoholics, and AIDS patients are typical examples of high-risk populations. Bacterial infections in the stomach other than *H. pylori* include other *Helicobacter* species, syphilitic gastritis, and tuberculosis. A small number of patients with dyspepsia harbor a spirochete-like organism named *H. heilmannii*. Prior domestic animal exposure may be a risk factor for such infections. AIDS patients are susceptible to developing overwhelming acute bacterial infection leading to the life-threatening phlegmonous gastritis. Gastric tuberculosis can also be seen in patients with AIDS. Syphilitic gastritis is a manifestation of the generalized mucocutaneous involvement of secondary syphilis.

Table 8.6 Other gastric infections

Causes	Organism
Bacterial, other than *Helicobacter pylori*	other *Helicobacter* spp. (e.g. *H. heilmannii*)
	phlegmonous gastritis
	tuberculosis
	syphilitic gastritis
Viral	cytomegalovirus
	herpes simplex virus
Fungal	cryptococcosis
	candidiasis
	histoplasmosis
Parasitic	giardiasis
	cryptosporidiosis
	strongyloides
	hookworm
	Anisakis spp.
	ascariasis

Cytomegalovirus gastritis is the most common viral gastritis, usually seen in the AIDS population or patients with other types of immunodeficiency. In children, CMV gastritis leads to a type of protein-losing enteropathy, the so-called childhood Menetrier disease. Rarely, HSV infection can lead to gastric mucosal erosions.

Parasitic gastritis usually occurs in the setting of high gastric pH. Helminthic infection by *Anisakis* spp. from eating raw fish is well recognized. Ascariasis, strongyloidiasis, and hookworm infections have also been reported. Gastric involvement of *Giardia* spp. and *Cryptosporidium* spp. is not uncommon among AIDS patients.

Finally, fungal infections such as histoplasmosis, cryptococcosis, and candidiasis have been reported, again primarily among AIDS or other immunodeficient patients.

Besides gastritis related to gastric infections, there are a number of other types of chronic gastritis (Box 8.3). These include sarcoidosis, lymphocytic gastritis (often associated with celiac sprue), eosinophilic gastroenteritis, hypertrophic gastropathy (adult Menetrier's disease), atrophic gastritis, and Crohn's disease.

Box 8.3 Non-infectious causes of gastritis

Sarcoidosis
Lymphocytic gastritis (sprue)
Eosinophilic gastroenteritis
Hypertrophic gastropathy (adult Menetrier's disease)
Atrophic gastritis
Crohn's disease

Further reading

Calam J. *Clinicians guide to Helicobacter pylori*. London: Chapman & Hall; 1996.

El-Omar EM, Penman ID, Ardill JES, Chittajallu RS, Howie C, McColl KEL. *Helicobacter pylori* infection and abnormalities of acid secretion in patients with duodenal ulcer disease. *Gastroenterology* 1995; 109: 681.

Harris AW, Grummett PA, Misiewicz JJ, Baron JH. Eradication of *Helicobacter pylori* in patients with duodenal ulcers lowers basal and peak acid outputs in response to gastrin releasing peptide and pentagastrin. *Gut* 1996; 38: 663.

Logan RPH, Walker MM, Misiewicz JJ, Gummett PA, Karim QN, Baron JH. Changes in the intragastric distribution of *Helicobacter pylori* during treatment with omeprazole. *Gut* 1995; 36: 12.

Vaira D, Malfertheiner P, Megraud F, *et al*. Diagnosis of *Helicobacter pylori* infection with a new non-invasive antigen-based assay. *Lancet* 1999; 354: 30–33.

Saponin P, Hyvarinen H, Psoralea M. *Helicobacter pylori* corpus gastritis relation to acid output. *J Physiol Pharmacol* 1996; 47: 151–159.

Laine L, Estrada R, Trujillo M, *et al*. Effect of proton-pump inhibitor therapy on diagnostic testing for *Helicobacter pylori*. *Ann Intern Med* 1998; 129: 547–550.

Lee J, O'Morain C. Who should be treated for *Helicobacter pylori* infection? A review of consensus conferences and guidelines. *Gastroenterology* 1997; 113 (Suppl): S99.

De Boer WA, Driessen WMM, Jansz AR, Tytgat GNJ. Effect of acid suppression on efficacy of treatment of *Helicobacter pylori*. *Lancet* 1995; 345: 817–820.

Walsh JH, Peterson WL. The treatment of *Helicobacter pylori* infection in the management of peptic ulcer disease. *N Engl J Med* 1995; 333: 984.

Hopkins RJ, Girardi LS, Turney EA. Relationship between *Helicobacter pylori* eradication and reduced duodenal and gastric ulcer recurrence: A review. *Gastroenterology* 1996; 110: 1244.

Uemura N, Okamoto S, Yamamoto S, *et al*. *Helicobacter pylori* infection and the development of gastric cancer. *N Engl J Med* 2001; 345(11): 784–789.

Laine L, Schoenfeld P, Fennerty MB. Therapy for *Helicobacter pylori* in patients with nonulcer dyspepsia. A meta-analysis of randomized, controlled trials. *Ann Intern Med*. 2001; 134(5): 361–369.

Montalban C, Santon A, Boixeda D, Bellas C. Regression of gastric high grade mucosa associated lymphoid tissue (MALT) lymphoma after *Helicobacter pylori* eradication. *Gut* 2001 49(4): 584–587.

Lee A, O'Rourke J. Gastric bacteria other than *Helicobacter pylori*. *Gastroenterol Clin North Am* 1993; 22: 21–42.

Chapter 9

Peptic Ulcer Disease

David C. Metz and Yu-Xiao Yang

CHAPTER OUTLINE

Introduction

Peptic ulcer disease is a common digestive disorder. Men and women are at equal risk for developing peptic ulcer disease, the overall lifetime risk for both sexes being 10%. Peptic ulcer disease is uncommon in children but the risk increases with age. In fact, over 70% of all peptic ulcer disease cases occur in persons between the age of 25 and 64 according to the National Health Interview Survey (NHIS), a federal government-sponsored national database. The prevalence of peptic ulcer disease is higher among African Americans and Hispanics than in Caucasians, and this is probably related to socioeconomic differences rather than a true racial influence. Such differences among the different racial groups are diminishing, probably owing to the widespread use of potent acid suppressants and anti-*Helicobacter pylori* treatment. The incidence of uncomplicated peptic ulcer disease is declining in the US owing to several reasons, but the incidence of bleeding ulcer is unchanged (Table 9.1).

There are about 6.7 million prevalent cases of peptic ulcer disease in the US; this is equivalent to 2490 cases per 100 000 persons. The crude mortality rate of peptic ulcer disease based on Center for Disease Control (CDC)

Table 9.1 Trends of uncomplicated versus bleeding peptic ulcer disease in the US

Uncomplicated peptic ulcer disease	Bleeding peptic ulcer disease
Decreased incidence due to disappearance of *Helicobacter pylori* and its eradication Wide-spread use of acid-suppressing drugs Selective use of NSAIDs and use of COX II inhibitors Better management of ICU patients	Still a significant problem. Incidence remains about 50/100 000 Rebleeding rate after hemostasis remains 15–25% Mortality remains about 5–12% Most associated with NSAIDs

statistics in 1998 was 1.74 deaths per 100 000 persons.

Given the high prevalence of peptic ulcer disease, the associated costs are also great (Figure 9.1). The hospital inpatient service costs associated with peptic ulcer disease account for more than half of the total direct costs of peptic ulcer disease.

In this chapter, the pathogenesis, clinical manifestations, diagnosis, and management of peptic ulcer disease will be discussed. *Helicobacter pylori* gastritis is covered in detail in chapter 8.

Pathogenesis

Physiology of acid secretion

To understand the pathophysiology of peptic ulcer disease, it is important to review briefly the normal physiology of gastric–acid secretion and mucosal cytoprotection. Gastric acid is normally produced by the parietal cell in response to stimulation by one of three possible secretagogues. The most important secretagogue, histamine, is released by enterochromaffin-like (ECL) cells, which are found throughout the gastric mucosa. Lesser secretagogues involved in parietal-cell stimulation include the vagal neurotransmitter; acetylcholine, which mediates the cephalic phase of acid secretion; and gastrin, which is released from antral G cells in response to antral distension, a rise in gastric pH, and other stimuli. Acetylcholine and gastrin also act directly on ECL cells, and it is currently believed that the primary action of the latter two secretagogues in humans is indirect stimulation of the parietal cell via the ECL cell. Following acid secretion by the parietal cell, a negative-feedback loop is activated that inhibits acid secretion and restores homeostasis. Most of this negative feedback loop is due to a positive (stimulatory) effect on somatostatin-releasing D cells found within the gastric antrum and fundus. Somatostatin functions primarily as a paracrine inhibitor of antral G cells and fundal parietal and ECL cells. The feedback inhibition of acid production allows for controlled secretion of acid in the presence of appropriate stimuli, such as after food ingestion, with a reduction in secretion during periods when there is no buffering capacity in the stomach. Figure 9.2 provides a diagrammatic overview of the control of acid secretion in the normal individual.

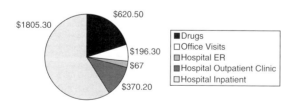

Figure 9.1 Direct costs of peptic ulcer disease (in millions).

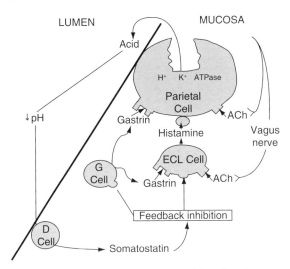

Figure 9.2 Gastric secretion and feedback.

Important factors on the cytoprotective side of the equation are mucosal bicarbonate and mucus secretion, as well as an increased submucosal blood delivery of protective factors such as prostaglandins or epidermal growth factor. Peptic ulcers develop when these homeostatic mechanisms become abnormal (Figure 9.3). Auto-digestion of the gastrointestinal mucosa by acid and activated pepsin is the final common pathway in the development of peptic ulceration. It is generally believed that excessive acid secretion is more important in the pathogenesis of duodenal ulcers, whereas deficient mucosal cytoprotection is more important in the pathogenesis of gastric ulcers. The pathogenesis of pre-pyloric ulcers appears to depend on both factors.

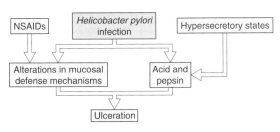

Figure 9.3 Pathogenesis of peptic ulcer disease.

Etiologic factors

Helicobacter pylori (see Chapter 8) and NSAID use remain the two leading causes of peptic ulcer disease. However, there are a number of other etiologic factors that need to be considered. Non-steroidal anti-inflammatory drug or aspirin use is the second leading cause of peptic ulcer disease, primarily gastric ulcers. The most widely used drugs are NSAIDs with more than 70 million prescriptions and more than 30 billion over-the-counter tablets sold annually in the US. More than 13 million Americans use NSAIDs daily, mostly for the treatment of joint inflammation. However, NSAID use is associated with adverse gastrointestinal events that pose significant limitations on the effectiveness of NSAIDs in the management of chronic arthritic diseases. In general, about 10% to 20% of patients have dyspepsia while taking NSAIDs. Furthermore, among chronic users, the annual incidence of serious gastrointestinal complications (perforations, bleedings, and symptomatic ulcers) is 1% to 4%. In the US, NSAID-induced gastrointestinal morbidity results in greater than 100 000 hospitalizations and 15 000 deaths annually.

Non-steroidal anti-inflammatory drugs and aspirin inhibit both cyclooxygenase-I and II (COX 1 and COX 2) (Figure 9.4). The proportion of COX 1 to COX 2 inhibition varies among different NSAIDs. It has been proposed that NSAIDs reduce inflammation and pain in patients with arthritis through inhibition of COX 2, an inducible enzyme that is stimulated by inflammation. On the other hand, NSAID-induced COX 1 inhibition leads to undesirable consequences, especially gastrointestinal mucosal damage by inhibiting the constitutively active COX isoform responsible for gastric mucosal cytoprotection. Normally, prostacyclin inhibits gastric-acid secretion, whereas prostaglandin E_2 and prostaglandin $F_{2\alpha}$ stimulate synthesis of protective mucus in the stomach and the

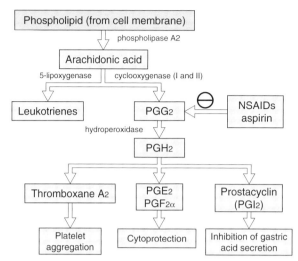

Figure 9.4 Arachidonic acid pathway. ⊖ = inhibits.

duodenum and thromboxane A_2 allows platelets to aggregate. Non-steroidal anti-inflammatory drugs and aspirin disable these protective mechanisms though the inhibition of COX 1 and COX 2. The resultant imbalance between acid secretion and diminished mucous protection leads to erosion, ulceration, and/or hemorrhage (Box 9.1).

COX 1 versus COX 2 inhibition

Based on the above paradigm, specific COX 2 inhibition should preserve the anti-inflammatory and analgesic effects of NSAIDs and at the same time cause little gastrointestinal toxic effects. In both animal and healthy volunteers, COX 2 inhibitors have been shown to

> **Box 9.1** Mechanisms of NSAID-induced gastric mucosal injury
>
> Decreased prostaglandin synthesis
> Altered protective mucus
> Increased acid back diffusion
> Decreased bicarbonate buffer
> Decreased gastric submucosal blood flow
> Direct epithelial injury

have anti-inflammatory effects with little gastrointestinal toxicity. More importantly, in clinical outcome trials, COX 2 inhibitors appear to be associated with a lower incidence of gastrointestinal complications in arthritis patients than non-selective NSAIDs, while preserving their anti-inflammatory capacity (Figure 9.5).

Interaction of *Helicobacter pylori* infection with NSAIDs

The prevalence of *Helicobacter pylori* infection among long- and short-term NSAID users is similar to that of the general population. In addition, *H. pylori* infection does not appear to worsen the degree of endoscopic mucosal injury associated with NSAID use. These data suggest that the ulcerogenic effects of NSAIDs and *H. pylori* infection are additive rather than synergistic, such that both etiologic agents need to be addressed independently. Recent work has shown that *H. pylori* infection can cause an up-regulation of gastric COX 2 expression and increase prostaglandin E_2 production. Cyclooxygenase II and its induction of mucosal prostaglandin E_2 are important in ulcer healing. It therefore is possible that *H. pylori* infection may be protec-

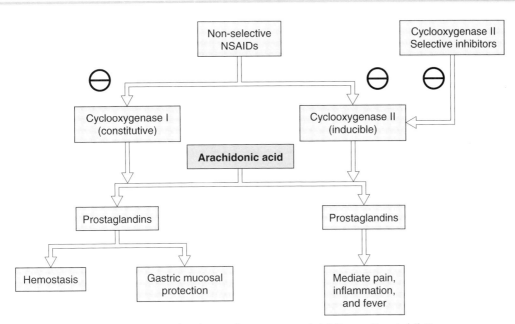

Figure 9.5 Selective versus non-selective cyclooxygenase inhibitors. ⊖ = inhibits.

tive against NSAID-related mucosal injury by promoting healing of ulcers that occur after NSAID exposure. In contrast, eradication of *H. pylori* infection before NSAID administration significantly reduced the occurrence of NSAID-related ulcers in one study. Other studies in chronic NSAID users have not revealed a benefit to *H. pylori* eradication.

Other etiologic factors

As suggested, the major environmental factors involved in the development of peptic ulcer disease are *Helicobacter pylori* gastritis and the use of NSAIDs. However, hypersecretory conditions, including Zollinger–Ellison syndrome, are less common but important causes. Other environmental influences that probably contribute more by preventing healing of ulcers rather than directly causing them include corticosteroid use, cigarette smoking, stress, and dietary factors including alcohol, coffee, and other substances. Peptic ulcers are also commonly associated with, but probably not directly caused by, certain medical conditions, including chronic obstructive pulmonary dis-

ease, ischemic heart disease and end-stage liver or kidney disease, among others.

Genetic factors probably exert little influence on the risk of peptic ulcer disease. However, a number of genetic syndromes have been strongly associated with peptic ulcers. These include

- the hereditary form of Zollinger–Ellison syndrome (i.e. the form that occurs in association with multiple endocrine neoplasia syndrome type 1)
- systemic mastocytosis
- C1 esterase deficiency (hereditary angioneurotic edema)
- Neuhauser's syndrome, which is an autosomal dominant disease characterized by essential tremor, congenital nystagmus, sleep disturbances, and duodenal ulcers
- Van Allen's type of amyloidosis, characterized by amyloidosis of peripheral nerves and kidneys in association with duodenal ulcers
- the pachydermoperiostosis syndrome
- the leukonychia–gallstone–ulcer syndrome.

Box 9.2 lists the etiologic factors involved in the development of peptic ulcers, divided into genetic and environmental factors.

Box 9.2 Etiologic factors in peptic ulcer disease

Genetic influences
blood group O
hyperpepsinogenemia
genetic syndromes
multiple endocrine neoplasia type 1 with
  Zollinger–Ellison syndrome
C1-esterase deficiency
Neuhauser's syndrome
Van Allen's amyloidosis
pachydermoperiostosis
leukonychia–gallstones–ulcer syndrome
other undefined hereditary factors (e.g. twin
  studies)

Environmental influences
Helicobacter pylori gastritis
NSAIDs
sporadic Zollinger–Ellison syndrome
other hypersecretory states (e.g. idiopathic
  hypersecretion and systemic mastocytosis)
miscellaneous (e.g. corticosteroids, smoking,
  stress, dietary factors, co-morbid conditions)

Table 9.2 Sporadic versus hereditary Zollinger–Ellison syndrome (ZES) with multiple endocrine neoplasia type 1 (MEN-1)

Hereditary ZES	Sporadic ZES
25% of cases	75% of cases
Younger age group	Older age group
Often multiple tumors	Often single tumor
Associated with MEN-1	Not associated with MEN-1
Not surgically curable	Surgically curable

There are two forms of Zollinger–Ellison syndrome: a hereditary form and a sporadic form (Table 9.2). Hereditary Zollinger–Ellison syndrome is associated with multiple endocrine neoplasia type 1, which is an autosomal dominant disorder characterized by tumors of the pituitary (e.g. prolactinoma, Cushing's disease), and the pancreas (Zollinger–Ellison syndrome, pancreatic polypeptidoma, and others), as well as four-gland parathyroid hyperplasia.

Zollinger–Ellison syndrome is a rare condition (incidence less than 1 per million) characterized by severe gastric-acid hypersecretion, peptic ulceration, and a non-beta islet-cell tumor. This syndrome was first described in 1955 by Zollinger and Ellison. Disease results from inappropriate hypersecretion of gastrin by a neuroendocrine tumor, also referred to as a gastrinoma because of its hormonal product. Gastrinomas are virtually always located in the proximal duodenum or head of the pancreas in an area called the gastrinoma triangle. The gastrinoma triangle is defined by the junction of the cystic and common hepatic ducts superiorly, the junction of the second and third portions of the duodenum inferiorly, and the junction of the head and neck of the pancreas medially. Occasionally, gastrinomas arise in areas outside the gastrinoma triangle (ovarian and cardiac primaries have been described). The tumor releases gastrin in an uncontrolled manner, resulting in inappropriate hypersecretion of gastric acid.

Clinical presentation

Most patients with peptic ulcers have abdominal pain or dyspepsia. Dyspepsia is defined as upper abdominal pain or discomfort that is episodic or persistent and often associated with belching, bloating, heartburn, nausea, or vomiting. Occasionally, patients have asymptomatic ulcers that are found routinely during upper endoscopy or on X-ray. Some asymptomatic patients ultimately present with ulcer complications such as hemorrhage, perforation, or gastric-outlet obstruction. It has been said that these presentations are more common in the elderly and in patients with Zollinger–Ellison syndrome. Typically, the characteristics of the abdominal pain differ between duodenal and gastric ulcers (Table 9.3). However, it must be stressed that one cannot diagnose the location of a peptic ulcer or, for that matter, whether an ulcer is present at all by the pattern of the

Table 9.3 Comparison of clinical features of duodenal and gastric ulcers

	Duodenal Ulcer	Gastric Ulcer
Quality	dull and gnawing	
Location	epigastrium radiating to the back in a quarter of cases	epigastrium
Timing	occurring hours after eating awakening patients at night	occurring soon after eating
Inciting or relieving factors	relieved with food	precipitated by eating
Complications	hemorrhage perforation gastric outlet obstruction	
Extra-intestinal symptoms (e.g. in ZES/MEN-1)	hyperparathyroidism pituitary tumor syndromes renal stones lipomata	none
Physical examination	generally normal occasional non-specific epigastric tenderness weight loss in benign or malignant gastric ulcer weight gain in a few duodenal ulcer patients	
Differential diagnosis	gastroesophageal reflux disease gastroduodenal carcinoma or lymphoma Crohn's disease biliary disease pancreatic disease motility disorder infectious process musculoskeletal pain syndrome pleural effusion myocardial infarction pericarditis abdominal aortic aneurysm functional or non-ulcer dyspepsia	

ZES Zollinger–Ellison syndrome; MEN-1 multiple endocrine neoplasia type 1

dyspepsia. Symptoms of gastric-acid hypersecretion, especially diarrhea, should raise the suspicion of Zollinger–Ellison syndrome or another hypersecretory condition. Similarly, the presence of a positive family history of peptic ulcer disease (or associated features of the various hereditary syndromes) should raise the possibility of multiple endocrine neoplasia type 1 or other hereditary peptic ulcer syndromes.

Except for the rare situations in which peptic ulcers are associated with specific extra-intestinal manifestations, the physical examination in patients with uncomplicated gastric and duodenal ulcers is generally normal. Weight loss can occur in patients with either benign or malignant gastric ulcers, and weight gain can occur in patients with benign duodenal ulcers. As mentioned, epigastric tenderness is occasionally present, but it is a non-specific finding.

Peptic ulcers must be differentiated from other causes of dyspepsia (Table 9.3). The epigastrium is the typical location for referral of pain from any inflammatory process arising in the embryonic foregut. Thus, the differential diagnosis of peptic ulcer disease of the stomach and duodenum includes acid peptic disease of the esophagus (GERD); other gastroduodenal syndromes, including carcinoma, lymphoma, and Crohn's disease (which may present with ulceration); hepatobiliary disease; pancreatic disease; and functional bowel disease, as well as non-gastrointestinal conditions.

Diagnosis

Because of the non-specific nature of the symptoms of peptic ulcer disease, and because ulcers are commonly asymptomatic or present with complications, the initial approach to the management of patients with dyspepsia in modern clinical practice has evolved into determining whether or not the dyspepsia is due to the presence of an ulcer (i.e. ulcer dyspepsia versus non-ulcer dyspepsia). As suggested earlier, however, diagnosing a gastric or duodenal ulcer is, in itself, only part of the

diagnostic process. It is also important to diagnose the underlying cause of the ulcer so that appropriate therapy can be instituted to prevent recurrent disease.

Two methods are available for the anatomic diagnosis of peptic ulcer disease (Table 9.4). Barium radiography is inexpensive and safe. However, its sensitivity for the diagnosis of duodenal ulcers or small gastric ulcers is much lower than that of endoscopy. Upper gastrointestinal endoscopy is generally safe and highly sensitive for the diagnosis of peptic ulcer disease, especially duodenal ulcers. Endoscopy also allows the gastroenterologist to visually inspect the mucosa, obtain biopsies for rapid urease testing and histological examination, and measure gastric juice pH. However, it is more expensive than radiography. One area where barium radiography may be superior to endoscopy is in the diagnosis of linitis plastica. Thus barium radiography and endoscopy should be considered complementary in such situations.

Once an ulcer has been detected, it is important to attempt to make a causative diagnosis so that appropriate therapy can be instituted. The following algorithm (Figure 9.6) illustrates one systematic way of identifying and treating the underlying etiology of the ulcer.

The diagnosis of *Helicobacter pylori* gastritis may be made using invasive or non-invasive

	Advantages	Disadvantages
Endoscopy	Excellent sensitivity for peptic ulcer disease (92%). Superior to radiography for duodenal ulcers. Allows direct inspection. Allows biopsy. Better for distinguishing benign from malignant ulcers.	May miss linitis plastica. Higher cost.
Radiography	Superior to endoscopy for early linitis plastica. Lower cost.	May not be cost-effective if upper endoscopy is needed later on. Low sensitivity especially for small lesions (54%).

Table 9.4 Comparison of endoscopic and radiographic diagnostic modalities

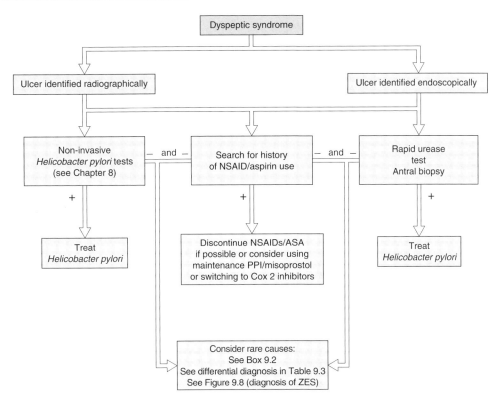

Note: NSAIDs and *Helicobacter pylori* infection can co-exist. Both need to be considered in all patients with ulcers.

Figure 9.6 Systematic way of identifying and treating the underlying etiology of peptic ulcer.

methods (see Chapter 8). The diagnosis of NSAID-induced ulcers is often made by exclusion in a patient with a positive history for NSAID use. Patients with arthritic complaints or chronic headaches commonly take large doses of NSAIDs for symptom relief without being aware of the risks of this behavior. This is especially important in elderly patients with arthritis. It is important to question patients very carefully about NSAID use. However, many studies have shown that direct questioning for the presence of prior NSAID use is often unhelpful in making a diagnosis. The utility of serum salicylate levels is debatable and probably not useful. As mentioned, patients undergoing endoscopy should have an antral biopsy performed if an ulcer is identified. The typical histologic finding in patients with NSAID-induced peptic ulcers is the absence of an inflammatory infiltrate.

Consequently, if a patient suspected of having a non-steroidal-induced ulcer is found to have significant inflammation on endoscopic antral biopsy, other causes (especially *H. pylori* gastritis) should be considered.

An important clue to the diagnosis of Zollinger–Ellison syndrome is an *H. pylori*-negative duodenal ulcer in a patient who does not use NSAIDs. In addition, Zollinger–Ellison syndrome should be considered in all patients with atypical duodenal ulcers (atypical by location or number), recurrent ulcers, ulcers associated with symptoms of gastric-acid hypersecretion, and ulcers associated with signs or symptoms compatible with multiple endocrine neoplasia syndrome type 1 (i.e. hyperparathyroidism, pituitary tumor syndromes, renal stones, lipomata, or a family history of such conditions). The diagnosis of Zollinger–Ellison syndrome depends on a combination of criteria, including fasting serum hypergastrinemia, elevated gastric–acid output measurements, positive provocative testing with secretin stimulation or calcium infusion, and, ultimately, by identification of a gastrinoma tumor. The initial screening test in all patients should be a fasting serum gastrin determination during a period when the patient is known to be producing gastric acid (i.e. in the absence of all anti-secretory medications, at least briefly).

Discontinuation of anti-secretory therapy (even for brief periods in a controlled setting) should not be undertaken without confirmation of ulcer healing as serious complications can result. A diagnostic approach (Figure 9.7) for Zollinger–Ellison syndrome is illustrated in the following flow chart.

Box 9.3 lists the causes of hypergastrinemia and divides them into those that are appropriate or physiologic and those that

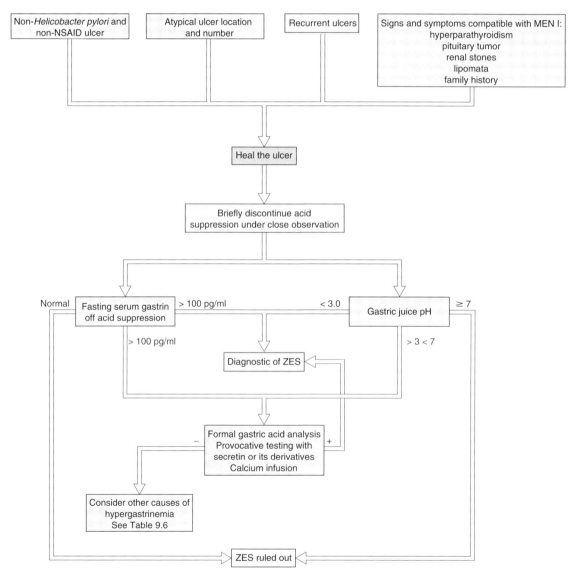

Figure 9.7 Diagnostic algorithm for Zollinger–Ellison syndrome (ZES). MEN-1 multiple endocrine neoplasia type 1.

> **Box 9.3** Causes of hypergastrinemia
>
> **Associated with hypo/achlorhydria (appropriate)**
> antisecretory therapy (histamine H_2-receptor antagonists or proton pump inhibitors)
> vagotomy (with or without gastric resection)
> atrophic gastritis (with or without pernicious anemia)
> *Helicobacter pylori* gastritis (pangastritis)
> chronic renal failure (common)
>
> **Associated with hyperchlorhydria (inappropriate)**
> Zollinger–Ellison syndrome
> antral G-cell hyperplasia/hyperfunction
> retained antrum syndrome
> chronic renal failure (rare)
> *Helicobacter pylori* gastritis (antral infection)
> gastric outlet obstruction (responds to decompression)
> small bowel resection (transient)

are inappropriate or pathologic. The latter causes of hypergastrinemia are generally distinguished from Zollinger–Ellison syndrome on clinical grounds, but all can cause ulcer disease.

Mastocytosis, hereditary angioneurotic edema, and other rare causes of peptic ulcer disease are generally diagnosed on the basis of their clinical presentation with or without specific blood tests (e.g. serum histamine levels, pepsinogen levels, etc.). Idiopathic hypersecretion is suspected in patients with ulceration associated with symptoms of gastric hypersecretion (i.e. diarrhea) and is confirmed by the presence of an elevated basal acid output (over 10 mEq/h) in the presence of a normal serum gastrin level (less than 100 pg/ml).

Management

The management of peptic ulcer disease can be divided into three broad categories:
1. healing the ulcer using medical and/or surgical therapy

2. treating the underlying cause of the ulcer to prevent recurrence, using antibiotics, antisecretory therapy, mucosal protectants, and surgery
3. treating ulcer complications.

Healing the ulcer

A number of medications are available for the healing of peptic ulcers. The advantages and disadvantages of each class of anti-ulcer medications are listed in Table 9.5.

Refractory ulcers

The proportion of ulcers that remain unhealed after standard courses of anti-ulcer therapy is inversely related to the length of therapy. Duodenal ulcers are considered refractory if healing is incomplete after 8 weeks of therapy. The response for gastric ulcers is somewhat slower than for duodenal ulcers, so that gastric ulcers are said to be refractory if healing is not complete by 12 weeks of therapy.

Several factors may delay healing and therefore render peptic ulcers refractory to treatment (Box 9.4). Among these, non-compliance is a major problem and should be sought for carefully.

Possible therapeutic approaches in patients with refractory ulcers are listed in Box 9.5.

Treating the underlying cause of the ulcer

The treatment of *Helicobacter pylori* infection is discussed in the prior chapter. The obvious approach to preventing recurrent ulcers in patients taking NSAIDs is to discontinue the drugs. Many patients who present with NSAID-induced ulcers are young, healthy people who have been taking them for self-limited conditions such as chronic headaches, menstrual cramps, or even peptic ulcer pain.

Table 9.5 Medications for peptic ulcer disease.

Medication	Pros	Cons	Comments
Antacids	More effective than placebo.	Metal content not appropriate for long-term therapy. Frequent doses required. Not very effective in relieving symptoms.	Not first-line therapeutic choice. Impractical.
Sucralfate	More effective than placebo. Comparable efficacy to H$_2$RAs.	Interfering with absorption of other medications. Poor compliance. Multiple doses required. Aluminum absorption a concern in renal patients	Not first-line therapeutic choice. Impractical.
H$_2$-receptor antagonists	90% healing after 8 weeks of therapy. Track record of efficacy and safety.	Gynecomastia in high doses (cimetidine). Interaction with cytochrome p450 enzymes. Requires renal dosing changes. Tolerance. Rebound hypersecretion (mild). Some gastric ulcers require more than 12 weeks of treatment.	Effective in almost all patients.
Proton pump inhibitors	More effective and more rapid healing. IV form available for ZES ulcers and bleeding ulcers.	Less interaction with cytochrome p450 enzymes. Non-specific GI symptoms, e.g. diarrhea.	Effective in most H$_2$RA-refractory ulcers. First line choice. Useful for anti-*Helicobacter pylori* therapy as well.
Prosta-glandins	Comparable effectiveness to H$_2$RA at high (ulcer-healing) doses. Effective in prevention of NSAID ulcers.	Frequent GI side effects, e.g. abdominal pain, diarrhea. Inappropriate in women of childbearing age.	Not first-line therapeutic choice. Impractical.
Anti-*Helicobacter pylori* antibiotics	Significantly decreases recurrence rates after successful eradication. More rapid healing with effective eradication.	Allergy. *Clostridium difficile* colitis.	Proven utility in ulcer dyspepsia.
Other agents carbenoxolone colloid bismuth anticholinergics	All have shown limited efficacy in healing peptic ulcers. Colloid bismuth is not available in the US.	Carbenoxolone and anti-cholinergics are associated with significant side effects.	Of historical interest only.

ZES Zollinger–Ellison Syndrome

Box 9.4 Causes of refractory ulcers

Poor compliance
NSAID use
Active cigarette smoking
Undiagnosed hypersecretory states
Persistent *Helicobacter pylori* gastritis
Other diseases masquerading as peptic ulcers
  (Crohn's disease, malignancy, eosinophilic
  gastroenteritis, etc.)

Box 9.5 Treatment options for refractory ulcers

Continuing treatment with H_2RA for a longer
  course or at higher doses
Changing to a different class of medications
  (i.e. proton pump inhibitors)
Using combination therapy with antibiotics if
  Helicobacter pylori gastritis is present
Substitution of a cytoprotective compound
  such as misoprostol or replacement of
  NSAIDs with COX II inhibitors in
  NSAID-dependent patients
Search for hypersecretory states and treat if
  positive
Anti-ulcer surgery (last resort in the modern
  era)

In these patients, substitution with other analgesics, such as acetaminophen, may be all that is required to prevent ulcer recurrence.

There is a group of patients, however, who are truly NSAID-dependent. These tend to be elderly people, often women, with severe arthritis. In these cases, prudent clinical management dictates that the smallest effective dose of NSAID be used and that therapy be taken with meals. Acute healing of NSAID-induced ulcers is more rapid if the NSAID is discontinued during therapy, although this is not essential and truly dependent patients can continue therapy along with proton pump inhibitors. Selective COX 2 inhibitors have been shown to have an equivalent efficacy in controlling pain as NSAIDs, but with a more favorable side-effect profile, i.e. a significantly improved ulcer rate. In addition, eradication of *H. pylori* may reduce the risk of ulceration from subsequent NSAID use in patients with minimal prior exposure to NSAIDs.

Misoprostol (at a dose of 200 µg q.i.d.) is the only drug currently approved for the prevention of NSAID-induced gastric ulcers. Misoprostol is also probably effective in preventing NSAID-induced duodenal ulcers. Diarrhea and abdominal cramps limit patient compliance, but these side effects are decreased if therapy is reduced to 100 µg q.i.d.. This lower-dose regimen, however, is less effective in preventing ulcers. Full doses of histamine H_2-receptor antagonists can prevent endoscopic duodenal ulceration from NSAIDs but

may not be effective in preventing gastric ulcers. Proton pump inhibitor maintenance is as effective as misoprostol for duodenal ulcers and better for gastric ulcers in terms of ulcer healing and relapse prevention.

Zollinger–Ellison syndrome

The initial approach to therapy in patients with Zollinger–Ellison syndrome is to manage the gastric-acid hypersecretion in order to prevent the development of complications. Thereafter, attention can be turned to identifying the location of the primary tumor, determining whether the disease is sporadic or associated with multiple endocrine neoplasia type 1 and, finally, determining whether the tumor is surgically resectable. The following flow chart (Figure 9.8) depicts a guideline for the acute and chronic management of Zollinger–Ellison syndrome patients.

By the time they present for medical care, patients with Zollinger–Ellison syndrome are often extremely ill and have life-threatening gastric-acid hypersecretion. Proton pump inhibitors are used as the mainstay of medical therapy for control of gastric-acid hypersecretion. Intravenous pantoprazole is highly effective in controlling acid output in patients with

Zollinger–Ellison syndrome. The dose approved by the Food and Drug Administration (FDA) for the use of this drug is 80 mg b.i.d. although 80 mg t.i.d. is required to control acid output in all patients. Intravenous pantoprazole represents a significant advance over continuous infusion H_2-receptor antagonists, the prior mainstay of therapy in patients with hypersecretory conditions who were unable to take oral therapy.

Once patients are able to take oral medication, they should be switched to oral anti-secretory therapy. Proton pump inhibitors are extremely potent anti-secretory agents with a long duration of action, such that acid output can be controlled in virtually all Zollinger–Ellison syndrome patients with once or twice daily dosing schedules without the development of tolerance.

Other agents are not generally used for the medical management of patients with Zollinger–Ellison syndrome because they are either ineffective or difficult to administer. An exception to this rule is the use of the somatostatin analogue, octreotide, which can be given two or three times daily by subcutaneous injection to control acid output and also reduce serum gastrin levels. There are also sustained-release formulations of octreotide available such as Depofoam® (SkyePharma, London) and long-acting repeatable (LAR®, Novartis, Basel, Switzerland), whose activity lasts 28 days. These formulations have good therapeutic efficacy and tolerability. Surgical control of gastric-acid hypersecretion is no longer the mainstay of treatment in patients with Zollinger–Ellison syndrome, because the available medical management is extremely effective. There is a role, however, for parathyroidectomy in patients with multiple endocrine neoplasia syndrome type 1. The coexistence of the hypercalcemia of hyperparathyroidism and the hypergastrinemia of Zollinger–Ellison syndrome exacerbates gastric-acid hypersecretion, and parathyroidectomy significantly reduces acid output in these patients. Total gastrectomy should be reserved only for the occasional patient who will not or cannot take oral medication.

Following the initial control of gastric-acid output, attention should be turned to defining the extent of the underlying disease and to determining whether the patient is potentially curable with surgery. Imaging studies, including magnetic resonance imaging, octreoscanning, endoscopic ultrasonography and secretin angiography, are important for identifying patients without obvious liver metastases who are surgical candidates, providing they have sporadic Zollinger–Ellison syndrome. It is important to distinguish multiple endocrine neoplasia type 1-associated Zollinger–Ellison syndrome from sporadic Zollinger–Ellison syndrome, because the hereditary form of the disease is not felt to be curable surgically. Patients with sporadic Zollinger–Ellison syndrome and localized disease on imaging studies should undergo exploratory laparotomy by an experienced surgeon, because about 34% to 40% of these patients can be cured surgically. Postoperative follow-up requires yearly monitoring with biochemical studies to confirm that there has not been a recurrence of Zollinger–Ellison syndrome that can lead to the development of severe recurrent gastric-acid hypersecretion.

Management of complications

Hemorrhage

Bleeding is the most common serious complication of peptic ulcer disease. It occurs in 15% to 20% of all patients. The mortality from peptic ulcer disease-associated bleeding remains as high as 10% in spite of newer hemostatic modalities. Patients with certain clinical features are more likely to have a poor prognosis (Box 9.6).

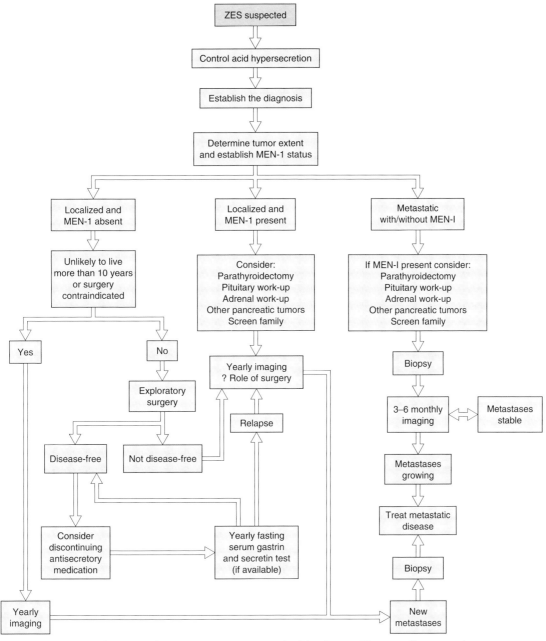

Figure 9.8 General approach to patients suspected of having Zollinger–Ellison syndrome (ZES). MEN-1 multiple endocrine neoplasia type 1.

The management of peptic ulcer disease bleeding begins with an initial phase of acute management followed by more definitive medical, endoscopic, and/or surgical treatment (Figure 9.9). Initial patient assessment should be carried out promptly based on the patient's vital signs and physical examination. Initial laboratory tests include complete blood count, coagulation times, type and cross-match. Resuscitation measures should be instituted immediately, usually with crystalloid solution via large-bore intravenous access. Urine output

> **Box 9.6** Predictors of poor outcome in patients with peptic ulcer disease-associated hemorrhage
>
> Large volume hematemesis
> Blood-tainted nasogastric aspirate not cleared after 6 liters of lavage
> Presence of shock on presentation
> Age over 60 years
> Presence of four or more pre-existing medical illnesses
> NSAID use

should be monitored closely to assess the patient's response to ongoing resuscitation efforts.

Once these emergency measures have been taken a nasogastric tube is placed. Nasogastric-tube aspirate can provide valuable information about the severity and acuity of the hemorrhage (Figure 9.9). Nasogastric lavage can also help clear the stomach to facilitate subsequent endoscopic examination and treatment. Endoscopy is potentially both diagnostic (i.e. rules out other causes of bleeding) and therapeutic (in high-risk lesions). The endoscopic appearance of identified lesions allows the endoscopist to predict the likelihood of recurrent bleeding and the need for intervention (Table 9.6).

If a patient develops recurrent bleeding after endoscopic hemostatic treatment, repeat endoscopic treatment should be performed while the patient is being evaluated for potential surgical and/or interventional radiology treatment, because repeat endoscopic treatment has been shown to be effective in a significant proportion of these patients. However, if repeated endoscopic hemostasis fails, surgery is the next option in most patients in order to control bleeding.

Once initial hemostasis is achieved, acid-suppression therapy with proton pump inhibitors should be started to reduce the risk of rebleeding. Recent studies have shown that patients with bleeding ulcers tend to have hypersecretion of gastric acid. In addition, low gastric pH impairs clot formation and clot stability (Box 9.7). Numerous past studies with intermittent or continuous infusion of H_2-receptor antagonists and intermittent proton pump inhibitor therapy have failed to show efficacy. However, there now is a mounting body of evidence showing adjunctive efficacy of continuous infusion of high-dose proton pump inhibitor therapy in addition to endoscopic hemostasis in high-risk patients. Therefore, for lesions at high risk for rebleeding, intravenous proton pump inhibitors (e.g. pantoprazole 80 mg i.v.p. followed by 8 mg/h for up to 3 days) should be given to prevent rebleeding from peptic ulcer disease.

Perforation

Perforation is a major cause of peptic ulcer disease morbidity and mortality. It occurs more often with duodenal ulcers than with gastric ulcers. Patients with peptic ulcer disease perforation usually present with signs and symptoms of an acute abdomen unless the perforation is retroperitoneal. In two thirds of the patients, a history of chronic peptic ulcer disease can be elicited. Most patients report sudden onset of severe, localized epigastric pain. The focal pain then becomes more generalized as the patient develops peritonitis. By the time the patients are examined, they usually are tachycardic, sometimes hypotensive, and in severe distress. The physical examination typically reveals a rigid abdomen with absence of bowel sounds. An upright X-ray of the abdomen and lower chest may reveal free air under the diaphragm. However, only 65% of cases are accompanied by the presence of free air. Therefore, the absence of free air does not rule out a perforation. The management of peptic ulcer disease perforation is primarily surgical. Non-operative management may

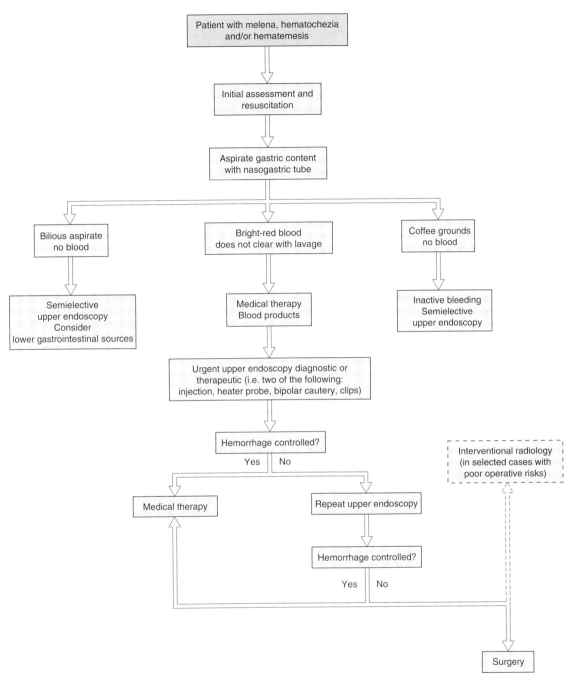

Figure 9.9 Management of acute upper gastrointestinal bleeding.

Table 9.6 The risk of rebleeding in various types of endoscopic lesions

Endoscopic appearance	Chance of rebleeding	Endoscopic intervention indicated
Active bleeding	80%	Yes
Visible vessel with no active bleeding	50%	Yes
Adherent clot	20%	No
Clear ulcer base	< 5%	No

Box 9.7 Rationale for Intravenous acid suppression therapy for peptic ulcer disease rebleeding prophylaxis

Gastric acid and pepsin inhibit clot formation
Gastric acid and pepsin cause clot lysis
Gastric acid impairs ulcer healing
Hypersecretion of gastric acid occurs in patients with ulcer bleeding

be considered in patients with prohibitive perioperative risks.

Gastric outlet obstruction

Gastric outlet obstruction is usually a consequence of chronic peptic ulcer disease, but it can also occur in patients with acute ulcers. Acute ulcers are associated with inflammation and local edema, which lead to pyloric stenosis. Chronic peptic ulcers cause gastric outlet obstruction through formation of scars and inflammation. Patients with gastric outlet obstruction present with early satiety, nausea, vomiting, bloating, reflux, and/or abdominal pain. Physical examination can sometimes reveal a succussion splash or a markedly distended stomach. X-ray studies may reveal a dilated stomach with a large air bubble. An upper gastrointestinal tract series can accurately delineate the nature of the stenosis, but if the barium does not pass this may hamper subsequent endoscopic attempts. Medical therapy consists of continuous nasogastric-tube decompression and healing the ulcer with proton pump inhibitors and *Helicobacter pylori* eradication when it is positive. Some patients may require endoscopic dilation to achieve symptomatic relief. Surgical treatment is reserved for those unresponsive to medical therapy.

Further reading

Chan FYK, Sung JJY, Chung SCS, *et al.* Randomised eradication of *Helicobacter pylori* before non-steroidal anti-inflammatory drugs therapy. To prevent peptic ulcer disease. *Lancet* 1997; 350: 975–979.

Collen MJ, Sheridan MJ. Definition for idiopathic gastric acid hypersecretion. *Dig Dis Sci* 1991; 36: 1371–1376.

Graham DY. The relationship between non-steroidal anti-inflammatory drug use and peptic ulcer. *Gastroenterol Clin North Am* 1990; 19: 171–182.

Hawkey CJ, Tulassay Z, Szcsepanski L, *et al.* Randomized controlled trial of *Helicobacter pylori* eradication in patients on non-steroidal anti-inflammatory drugs: HELP NSAIDs study. *Lancet* 1998; 352: 1016–1021.

Klinkenberg-Knol EC, Nelis F, Dent J, *et al.* Long-term omeprazole treatment in resistant gastroesophageal reflux disease: efficacy, safety and influences on gastric mucosa. *Gastroenterol* 2000; 118(4): 661–669.

Lam SK, Hui Wm, Ching CK. Peptic ulcer disease: epidemiology, pathogenesis, and etiology. In: Haubrich WB, Berk JE, Schaffner F (eds) *Bockus Gastroenterology*. Philadelphia PA: Saunders; 1994, 700–748.

Lamberts R, Creutzfeldt W, Struber HG, *et al.* Long-term omeprazole therapy in peptic ulcer disease: gastrin, endocrine cell growth and gastritis. *Gastroenterology* 1993; 104: 1356–1370.

Langman MJ, Jensen DM, Watson DJ, *et al.* Adverse upper gastrointestinal effects of Rofecoxib compared with NSAIDs. *JAMA* 1999; 282: 1929–1933.

Lew EA, Pisegna JR, Starr JA, *et al.* Intravenous pantoprazole rapidly controls gastric acid hypersecretion in patients with Zollinger–Ellison syndrome. *Gastroenterology* 2000; 118: 696–704.

Martin TR, Vennes JA, Silvis SE, Ansel HJ. A comparison of upper gastrointestinal endoscopy and radiography. *J Clin Gastroenterol* 1980; 2: 21–25.

Metz DC, Jensen RT. Endocrine tumors of the pancreas. In: Haubrich WB, Berk F, Schaffner JE (eds) *Bockus Gastroenterology*. Philadelphia PA: Saunders; 1994, 3002–3034.

Norton JA, Fraker DL, Alexander HR, *et al.* Surgery to cure the Zollinger–Ellison syndrome. *N Engl J Med* 1999; 341: 635–644.

Soll, AH, Weinstein, WM, Kurata, J, McCarthy, D. Non-steroidal anti-inflammatory drugs and peptic ulcer disease. *Ann Intern Med* 1991; 114: 307.

Chapter 10

Gastroparesis and Other Gastric Motor Abnormalities

Janak N. Shah and David C. Metz

CHAPTER OUTLINE

Introduction

Gastroparesis literally implies "gastric paralysis". It is defined as delayed emptying of ingested contents from the stomach into the duodenum that is attributed to disordered motility and is in the absence of anatomic obstruction. Gastroparesis can lead to upper gastrointestinal tract symptoms, such as nausea, vomiting, upper-abdominal pain, and bloating. Assessments of gastric emptying help for diagnosis and provide an important global indication of gastric motor function.

Recently, practitioners are increasingly recognizing patients with upper gastrointestinal symptoms attributed to gastric neuromuscular abnormalities in the setting of normal overall gastric emptying. Improved understanding and advances in technology have allowed us to characterize more subtle motor abnormalities such as antral hypomotility, impaired fundic relaxation, dyssynchronous antroduodenal coordination, pylorospasm, and gastric dysrhythmias.

Physiology

The stomach is designed to receive and store ingested material, prepare food for digestion by mixing with gastric secretions, grind solid food into small particles, and deliver nutrients into the small intestine for digestion. The proximal stomach is primarily involved with the storage of ingested food. Swallowing initiates a vagally mediated transient receptive relaxation of the fundus, which is followed by a more prolonged relaxation phase (accommodation) that occurs in response to gastric distension (mediated by gastric mechanoreceptors) as ingested food accumulates. This process allows for increases in gastric volume to accommodate eating without substantial increases in intragastric pressure.

The distal stomach (distal body and antrum) is responsible for breaking down and emptying food contents. Rhythmic contractions of the distal stomach are controlled by electrical signals (gastric slow waves) initiated from a pacemaker region (interstitial cells of Cajal) along the greater curvature in the proximal gastric body. Gastric slow waves occur at a frequency of 3 cycles per minute, and are propagated circumferentially and distally through smooth muscle layers. Whether gastric slow waves result in contractile activity in the distal stomach is determined by neural and hormonal influences. In general, fewer gastric slow waves lead to contractions in quiescent (fasting) states as compared to stimulated (postprandial) states.

Postprandially, ingested contents that are initially stored in the fundus empty at different rates depending on their composition. Non-nutrient liquids empty at linear rates, and depend on pressure differences between the proximal stomach and the pylorus or duodenum. The emptying of nutrient-rich liquids and digested or liquefied solids also follows a linear rate, but is primarily dependent on feedback from lumenal receptors in the small intestine. Specific receptors for nutrients such as glucose, fatty acids, and amino acids, help regulate gastric emptying rates through neurohormonal mechanisms. Of these, lipids are the strongest inhibitors of gastric emptying.

The gastric emptying rate for solids is characterized by a lag phase, during which ingested solid material is transferred from the proximal to distal stomach, where it is crushed into smaller particles by powerful antral contractions. Small particles that are less than 1 to 2 mm may then empty into the duodenum at a nearly linear rate of emptying. Although specific mediator pathways are unclear, postprandial gastric motility appears to be regulated by neurohormonal factors, and is influenced by vagal stimulation as well as hormones, such as gastrin, motilin, cholecystokinin, somatostatin, dopamine, glucagon, vasoactive intestinal peptide, and secretin. Other pathways that help regulate gastric motility involve dopaminergic (D_2), opiate, muscarinic, and serotinergic ($5-HT_3$ and $5-HT_4$) receptors.

In the fasting state, gastric motility is cyclical, and is composed of three phases with a cycle time of about 100 minutes. The cyclical pattern is known as the migrating motor complex. Phase I is a period of motor quiescence, and comprises the majority of the cycle length. Phase II contains increased, but infrequent and irregular, motor contractions. Phase III lasts for about 5 minutes and consists of regular, high-amplitude contractions at a rate of 3 per min. It is during this phase that particles of debris larger than 5 mm in size empty into the duodenum. This is often referred to as the "housecleaning" function of the migrating motor complex, and clears the gastrointestinal tract of non-digestible solids during the fasting state. Figure 10.1 illustrates components of normal postprandial and fasting gastric neuromotor physiology.

Normal gastric emptying involves a complex mechanism with different postprandial and fasting patterns, and is controlled by various neurohormonal pathways that are incompletely understood. Abnormalities at any stage may lead to gastroparesis, and may produce clinically significant symptoms.

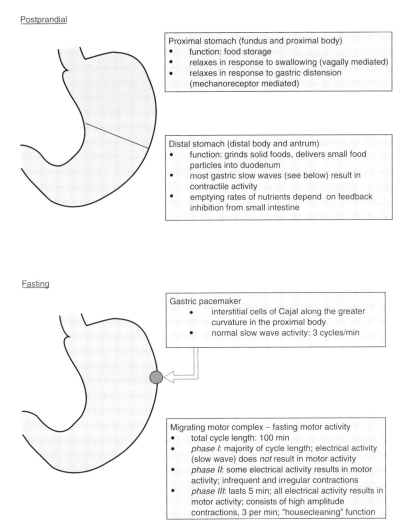

Postprandial

Proximal stomach (fundus and proximal body)
- function: food storage
- relaxes in response to swallowing (vagally mediated)
- relaxes in response to gastric distension
  (mechanoreceptor mediated)

Distal stomach (distal body and antrum)
- function: grinds solid foods, delivers small food
  particles into duodenum
- most gastric slow waves (see below) result in
  contractile activity
- emptying rates of nutrients depend on feedback
  inhibition from small intestine

Fasting

Gastric pacemaker
- interstitial cells of Cajal along the greater
  curvature in the proximal body
- normal slow wave activity: 3 cycles/min

Migrating motor complex – fasting motor activity
- total cycle length: 100 min
- *phase I*: majority of cycle length; electrical activity
  (slow wave) does *not* result in motor activity
- *phase II*: some electrical activity results in motor
  activity; infrequent and irregular contractions
- *phase III*: lasts 5 min; all electrical activity results in
  motor activity; consists of high amplitude
  contractions, 3 per min; "housecleaning" function

Figure 10.1 Normal, postprandial, and fasting gastric neuromotor physiology.

Etiology

Numerous diseases and conditions may lead to neuromuscular dysfunction and delay gastric emptying (Table 10.1). Anatomic obstruction may impede gastric emptying and should be investigated prior to considering gastroparesis. Gastroparesis is thus a diagnosis of exclusion, implying that structural obstruction had been ruled out with appropriate tests. Common causes of chronic delayed gastric emptying include diabetic, postsurgical, and idiopathic etiologies.

Although diabetic gastroparesis is typically seen in patients with long-standing type 1 disease (over 10 years), with complications of peripheral and autonomic neuropathy, it may be found in those with shorter duration of disease or in type 2 diabetics. The pathogenesis of diabetic gastroparesis appears to be linked to vagal neuropathy. Additionally, hyperglycemia plays an important role, with improvements in gastric emptying noted in diabetics during euglycemia. Interestingly, symptoms do not universally correlate to objective

Table 10.1 Etiology of gastroparesis*	
Major subtypes	Common examples
IDIOPATHIC	post-viral or truly idiopathic gastric resection with vagotomy
POST-SURGICAL	Roux-en-Y gastrojejunostomy, fundoplication, gastric bypass, esophagectomy, Whipple procedure, heart–lung transplant, postoperative ileus
MEDICATIONS	anticholinergics, beta-adrenergics, calcium channel blockers, opiates, levodopa, lithium, phenothiazine, progesterone, nicotine, alcohol, marijuana
Metabolic	**DIABETES**, hypothyroidism, hypokalemia, hyperglycemia, hypo or hypercalcemia, renal failure
Neurologic	Stroke, central nervous system, or spinal cord injury, brain tumors, seizures, migraines, Parkinson's disease, Guillain–Barré syndrome, multiple sclerosis
Psychiatric	Anorexia nervosa, bulimia, rumination syndrome
Oncologic	Paraneoplastic syndrome (breast, lung, pancreas cancer), post-radiation therapy, linitis plastica (diffusely infiltrating gastric adenocarcinoma), gastric lymphoma, abdominal malignancy associated
Rheumatologic	Scleroderma, systemic lupus erythematosus, polymyositis, dermatomyositis
Infectious	Epstein–Barr virus, varicella zoster, parvovirus-like, Chagas' disease, *Clostridium botulinum*, human immunodeficiency virus
Other	GERD-related, chronic intestinal pseudoobstruction, myotonic dystrophy, amyloidosis, eosinophilic gastroenteritis
* The most common causes are in bold, capital letters	

findings of gastroparesis. Some asymptomatic diabetics demonstrate abnormal emptying by scintigraphy, while others with severe nausea and vomiting may have normal gastric emptying studies. Such findings may be attributed to other types of gastric neuromuscular dysfunction, such as gastric dysrhythmias, in the setting of normal global emptying.

Postsurgical gastroparesis may develop following a variety of gastric, esophageal, and thoracic surgical procedures. Symptoms of gastroparesis may develop immediately postoperatively, or months or even years later, and the etiology must be distinguished from anatomic obstruction.

Idiopathic gastroparesis is defined as delayed gastric emptying without an apparent cause. It may be sudden in onset, or may present insidiously. A subset of patients with idiopathic gastroparesis report prodromal symptoms of fevers, myalgias, nausea, and diarrhea, suggestive of a viral etiology. But instead of self-limited symptoms of a viral illness, their symptoms of delayed gastric emptying last months to years before resolving, if they do resolve at all. Overall, patients with idiopathic gastroparesis attributed to a viral etiology report gradual improvement, while those without a viral prodrome report more progressive, chronic symptoms.

Many other rarer causes of gastroparesis exist. These include neuropsychiatric, oncologic, rheumatologic, metabolic, and infectious diseases (Table 10.1). Many medical and non-medical drugs may decrease gastric emptying. The more commonly implicated ones include calcium channel blockers, antidepressants, pain medications, nicotine, and alcohol. Some diseases have diffuse involvement and lead to altered motor activity in the entire gastrointestinal tract. These include amyloidosis, eosinophilic gastroenteritis, and connective tissue diseases such as scleroderma.

Non-ulcer dyspepsia and gastroparesis

Non-ulcer dyspepsia (or functional dyspepsia) refers to non-specific upper gastrointestinal symptoms in the absence of identifiable disease. Some patients who are classified as having non-ulcer dyspepsia may actually have delayed gastric emptying as a cause of symptoms. Therefore, tests of gastric emptying (see Diagnostic Studies, p. 154) should be performed in these patients prior to establishing the diagnosis of non-ulcer dyspepsia. However, the majority of these patients will have normal gastric emptying based on current studies (scintigraphy) that give estimates of global gastric motor activity. We must keep in mind that our present understanding of non-ulcer dyspepsia is in flux. Improvements and dissemination of diagnostic technology may soon allow us to recognize more subtle gastric motor and sensory abnormalities that we are currently classifying as non-ulcer dyspepsia, and may lead to new treatment approaches for this disease entity. Non-ulcer dyspepsia is discussed in detail in Chapter 11.

Table 10.2 Symptoms of gastroparesis (*n* = 146) (from Soykan I, Sivri B, Sarosiek I, *et al.* Demography, clinical characteristics, psychological and abuse profiles, treatment, and long-term follow-up of patients with gastroparesis. *Dig Dis Sci* 1998; 43(11): 2398, with permission)

Symptom	Percentage of patients
Nausea	92
Vomiting	84
Bloating	75
Early satiety	60
Abdominal pain	46

Clinical presentation

Symptoms of gastroparesis include chronic or intermittent nausea, vomiting, early satiety, bloating, belching, postprandial abdominal pain, weight loss, and gastroesophageal reflux symptoms (Table 10.2). All are symptoms that may be present with a variety of gastrointestinal disorders, and none is specific to gastric motor dysfunction. Patients with mild disease may only be symptomatic postprandially with improvement between meals, while patients with severe gastroparesis may constantly feel symptoms. Vomited contents are often characteristically composed of recognizable food residue that was ingested more than 8 to 12 hours previously. Patients with gastroparesis are at increased risk for developing bezoars. Worsening of symptoms over baseline, or new onset abdominal or back pain may suggest their presence.

No physical examination findings are specific for diagnosis. The presence of a succussion splash suggests inadequate gastric emptying, but may be present in either gastroparesis or mechanical obstruction. A succussion splash is best elicited by rocking the patient back and forth in an upright position while placing a stethoscope over the epigastrium. The movement of retained contents

Table 10.3 Diagnostic tests in the evaluation of gastroparesis		
Test	Advantages	Disadvantages
Structural		
Upper endoscopy	used to rule out mechanical obstruction, widely available, ability to biopsy lesion, no radiation	invasive
Contrast study	widely available	radiation exposure
Emptying		
Scintigraphy	widely available, accurate, non-invasive, easy to interpret	radioactive
Radiopaque markers	cheap, widely available	radiation, indirect reflection of emptying
Ultrasound	non-invasive, non-radiating	expensive, not widely available, requires interpretive expertise
Magnetic resonance imaging	non-invasive, non-radiating	expensive, not widely available, requires interpretive expertise
Epigastric impedance	non-invasive, non-radiating, cheap	movement artifact
^{13}C Octanoic acid breath test	non-invasive, non-radioactive, good correlation to scintigraphy	not widely available
Neuromuscular function		
Gastric manometry	measures fasting and postprandial motor activity	invasive, not widely available, requires interpretive expertise
Electrogastrogram	non-invasive, only test for gastric dysrhythmias	not widely available, requires interpretive expertise
Gastric barostat	Only test for measuring visceral hypersensitivity	invasive, not widely available

against the gastric wall will produce a characteristic "splash" sound that is audible with a stethoscope. Other examination findings may help reveal the etiology once gastroparesis is confirmed (e.g. malar rash for lupus, peripheral neuropathy for diabetes). Further diagnostic tests may be obtained depending on the specific underlying etiology that is suspected.

Diagnostic studies

Several diagnostic tests are available in the evaluation of gastroparesis (Table 10.3).

Structural studies

Most patients in whom gastroparesis is entertained should first undergo structural evaluation of the upper gastrointestinal tract to exclude mechanical obstruction. Commonly used tests include upper endoscopy and upper gastrointestinal contrast radiography. Both tests are important in the evaluation of these patients primarily to exclude other causes of gastrointestinal symptoms. However, they may reveal findings that are highly suggestive of delayed emptying. In fact, some advocate that findings of retained food following an 8-hour fast in the absence of obstruction is diagnostic of gastroparesis. Additionally, complete retention of barium at 30 minutes, or presence of any barium at 6 hours on upper gastrointestinal contrast radiography is considered abnormal. Although these studies may reveal findings that strongly support gastroparesis, nuclear scintigraphy remains the standard for diagnosis. Importantly, absence of food debris following a fast and normal emptying of barium does not exclude gastroparesis.

Nuclear scintigraphy

Nuclear scintigraphy is the most widely used modality to diagnose gastroparesis. It involves the scintigraphic assessment of gastric emptying using radiolabeled meals. Both solid- and liquid-phase emptying can be quantifiably measured. Liquid-phase emptying is usually performed with the aqueous isotope ^{111}indium-diethylenetramine pentacetic acid, which is ingested with water. Solid-phase scans usually involve ^{99m}technetium-sulfur colloid mixed with scrambled eggs. The egg meal is preferred because the radiotracer binds to egg albumin during cooking. As different radiotracers are used, both solid and liquid phases may be performed simultaneously. After meal ingestion, a gamma camera is placed over the abdomen to record radioactivity from the stomach at set intervals (usually every 15 to 30 min for 2 to 4 hours). Results are usually given as the percentage of the meal that is emptied at 2 hours, or the length of time for one half of the meal to empty. In normal patients, about 50% of a solid meal empties within 2 hours.

Solid-phase scans are more sensitive than liquid-phase scans for the diagnosis of gastroparesis, and are the preferred modality. Liquid-phase studies are only recommended in patients unable to tolerate solids, with symptoms that are only present during the ingestion of fluids (uncommon), and occasionally to confirm gastroesophageal reflux (although other much more sensitive tests of reflux exist).

Recent advances in technology now allow for the continuous assessment of gastric motility with scintigraphy. Such dynamic techniques may allow us to delineate regional intragastric movement patterns, and may help us characterize other gastric dysmotility states such as antral hypomotility. Currently these techniques are mostly used as research tools.

Other tests of emptying

Radiopaque markers may be used to assess gastric emptying. After ingestion, interval radiographs help estimate emptying time. No markers should remain in the stomach by 6 hours after ingestion. Because of their size, markers empty during phases II and III of the migrating motor complex. As emptying of these non-digestible markers depends on fasting motor activity, emptying rates are not direct reflections of postprandial gastric emptying, and their clinical relevance is questionable. This test is inexpensive, but involves radiation.

Ultrasonography and magnetic resonance imaging can be used to study gastric emptying. After ingestion of a liquid meal, serial ultrasound examinations may be performed over the antrum. Return to a fasting baseline antral area correlates to complete emptying. Advances in three-dimensional imaging should allow more accurate volumetric assessments, and allow us to characterize regional intragastric meal distribution. Unfortunately, solid meals cannot be assessed by ultrasound because of their echogenicity. Magnetic resonance imaging has been used in a similar fashion, and provides accurate volumetric measurements of gastric emptying. Rapid scan technology delineates regional intragastric wall motion. Advantages of these techniques include lack of radiation, but the disadvantages are that they are not widely available, are generally more expensive than scintigraphy, and are primarily used as research tools.

Epigastric impedance measures resistance to passage of electrical currents through the stomach using cutaneous electrodes. Ingestion of low conductivity liquid meals changes the resistance which can be serially measured to estimate gastric emptying. This test is subject to motion artifact and is not widely used. However, it is inexpensive, non-invasive, and radiation free.

Breath tests using ^{13}C-octanoic acid have shown good correlation with estimates of gastric emptying by scintigraphy. The test involves the measurement of $^{13}CO_2$ in the expired breath following ^{13}C-octanoic acid-labeled meal ingestion (solid or liquid). Reliable interpretation requires normal small intestinal absorption. This test may be especially useful in patients in whom radioactive tracers should be avoided (children and pregnant women). Although currently considered a research tool, ^{13}C-octanoic acid breath tests hold promise for future widespread use in the evaluation of gastroparesis.

Tests of neuromuscular function

Antroduodenal manometry studies are performed over at least 6 to 8 hours. Initially, fasting motility patterns of the migrating motor complex are recorded, followed by meal ingestion and evaluation of the postprandial pattern. An advantage of this technique is the ability to immediately test the response to prokinetic drugs. The technique has been useful to detect gastroparesis with decreased antral activity in fasting or postprandial states, pylorospasm, and dyssynchronous antroduodenal coordination. Smaller manometric catheters allow 24-hour ambulatory evaluations.

The electrogastrogram records electrical slow wave activity for the stomach, analogous to the electrocardiogram for the heart. Although electrogastrograms were initially done using serosal leads, advances in signal processing and computer analysis have allowed performance with cutaneous leads. Filtering techniques enable the selective evaluation of gastric electrical activity. Electrogastrograms should be performed under fasting and fed states, with the patient minimizing motion to avoid artifacts. Deviations from the normal 3 cycles per min establish the diagnoses of bradygastria (less than 2 cpm) or tachygastria (more than 4 cpm). Dysrhythmias are usually caused by ectopic gastric pacemakers. As not all gastric electrical activity corresponds to contractile activity, there is limited correlation between electrogastrogram results and gastric emptying. The current role for this test in clinical practice is not yet defined. None the less, electrogastrograms may become complimentary to emptying tests (scintigraphy), and together may become useful in connecting patient symptoms to abnormal gastric neuromotor physiology. Currently, this technique is limited to specialized centers with expertise in gastrointestinal motility.

Gastric barostat studies involve the placement of a balloon device in the stomach to assess visceral sensitivity to pressure and volume. The device can measure gastric tone and accommodation. The balloon is inflated to various pressures and volumes in different locations of the stomach to identify threshold values that lead to symptoms. This technique appears useful to characterize and localize visceral hypersensitivity. Currently, it is mainly used as a research tool.

Clincal evaluation

Figure 10.2 illustrates an algorithmic approach to the evaluation of a patient with suspected gastroparesis. The first step involves a structural study of the gastrointestinal tract (upper endoscopy or contrast radiography) to exclude a mechanical obstruction. Patients

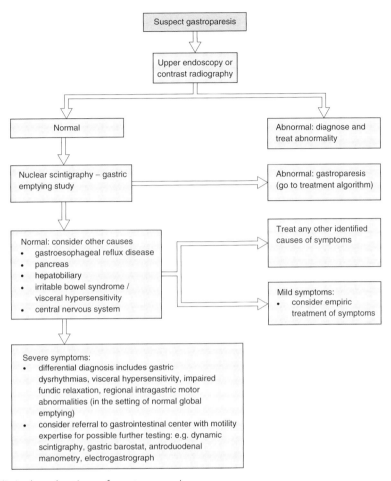

Figure 10.2 Clinical evaluation of gastroparesis.

with normal studies should then undergo nuclear gastric emptying scans. If abnormal, the diagnosis is confirmed. If normal, other atypical, non-gastric causes of symptoms should be considered (e.g. GERD, pancreatic and hepatobiliary causes). Additionally, one must realize that as gastric emptying studies measure global emptying, they may not recognize more subtle motor abnormalities, and are not useful to assess gastric sensory dysfunction (hypersensitivity). At this point, patients lacking a definite diagnosis, but with only mild discomfort, may be empirically treated for their symptoms. Lifestyle and dietary modifications, acid suppressants, and low-dose antidepressants (for visceral hypersen-

sitivity) should be considered. Patients with more severe, debilitating symptoms should be referred to gastrointestinal centers with expertise in motility abnormalities for further testing (e.g. dynamic scintigraphy, gastric barostat, gastric manometry).

Treatment

The treatment of gastroparesis can be quite challenging. The primary goal of treatment is to control symptoms. Patients with delayed gastric emptying, but no symptoms, do not require therapy other than that indicated for

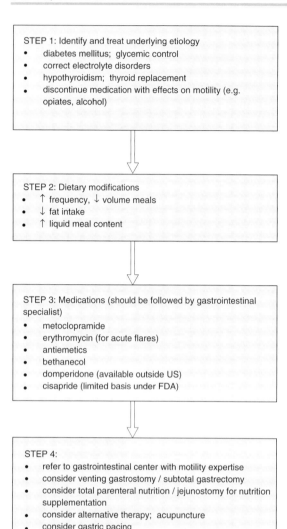

STEP 1: Identify and treat underlying etiology
- diabetes mellitus; glycemic control
- correct electrolyte disorders
- hypothyroidism; thyroid replacement
- discontinue medication with effects on motility (e.g. opiates, alcohol)

STEP 2: Dietary modifications
- ↑ frequency, ↓ volume meals
- ↓ fat intake
- ↑ liquid meal content

STEP 3: Medications (should be followed by gastrointestinal specialist)
- metoclopramide
- erythromycin (for acute flares)
- antiemetics
- bethanecol
- domperidone (available outside US)
- cisapride (limited basis under FDA)

STEP 4:
- refer to gastrointestinal center with motility expertise
- consider venting gastrostomy / subtotal gastrectomy
- consider total parenteral nutrition / jejunostomy for nutrition supplementation
- consider alternative therapy; acupuncture
- consider gastric pacing
- consider enrollment in trials of investigational drugs

Figure 10.3 Treatment of gastroparesis.

their underlying disease states (e.g. glucose control for diabetes).

First-line therapy involves the correction of underlying disorders that are causing or exacerbating the gastroparesis. Electrolyte abnormalities should be corrected, medications affecting motility should be discontinued, and metabolic abnormalities (diabetes, hypothyroidism) should be treated. Addressing underlying conditions may relieve symptoms. If unsuccessful, dietary modifications and medications should then be instituted.

Ultimately, patients with severe symptoms that are unresponsive to conservative measures may require surgical or other innovative approaches. Figure 10.3 illustrates a stepwise approach to therapy.

Dietary modifications

Liquids empty more readily than solids, so meals of higher liquid content are recommended. Fiber intake should be minimized as fiber delays gastric emptying and may lead to bezoar formation. Small-volume, frequent meals consisting of mechanically soft, low-fat content are suggested. In gastroparesis patients with significant nausea and vomiting, a stepwise approach to oral intake should begin with salty liquids (glucose electrolyte solutions or bouillon); followed by noodle soups, rice, and crackers; and finally include starches, chicken, and fish.

Prokinetic medications

Several prokinetic medications may be useful in the management of gastroparesis (Table 10.4). They vary in their mechanism of action, antiemetic properties, side effects, and market availability. There have been no large, comparative studies of these agents in gastroparesis patients. However, one meta-analysis suggested that metoclopramide provides the best symptom control, while erythromycin is the strongest stimulant for gastric emptying.

Metoclopramide

Metoclopramide has prokinetic actions via serotonin receptor ($5-HT_4$) facilitation of cholinergic stimulation, dopamine receptor (D_2) antagonism in the myenteric plexus, and direct smooth muscle contraction through sensitization of muscarinic receptors. There

Table 10.4 Commonly used prokinetic medications

Drug	Mechanism	Dosage	Side effects
Metoclopramide	5-HT$_4$ agonist, D$_2$ and 5-HT$_3$ antagonist	5–20 mg q.i.d. p.o./ i.v./i.m./s.c.	↑ prolactin, drowsiness, dystonia, tardive dyskinesia
Domperidone*	D$_2$ antagonist	10–30 mg q.i.d. p.o.	↑ prolactin
Cisapride**	5-HT$_4$ agonist, 5-HT$_3$ antagonist	10–20 mg b.i.d. to q.i.d., p.o.	abdominal cramping, diarrhea, ventricular arrhythmia
Bethanecol	Muscarinic agonist	25 mg q.i.d., p.o.	abdominal cramping, flushing, diaphoresis, nausea, vomiting
Erythromycin	Motilin agonist	50–200 mg q.i.d. p.o 1–2 mg/kg every 8 h, i.v.	abdominal cramping, nausea, vomiting, tachyphylaxis

*not FDA approved, available in non-US countries including Canada and Mexico.
**only available through limited access protocols directly from manufacturer under careful FDA scrutiny.

are additional antiemetic actions centrally through dopamine (D$_2$) and serotonin receptor (5-HT$_3$) antagonism of vagal and brainstem pathways. Specific neuromotor effects of metoclopramide in the stomach include increased antral contractions with decreased pyloroduodenal tone (improves antroduodenal coordination), and inhibition of fundic accommodation (promotes gastric emptying). It has minimal colonic effects. It has been used in the management of gastroparesis in diabetics and patients with prior gastric surgery, and is the only US FDA-approved agent for diabetic gastroparesis.

As the onset of action is within 1 hour of an oral dose, the medication is usually taken half an hour before meals. Usual doses range from 5 to 20 mg taken four times daily. Side effects occur in up to 15% to 20% of patients, and commonly include drowsiness, agitation, and dystonic reactions. Dystonic reactions may include involuntary movements, facial grimacing, torticollis, tongue protrusion, and trismus. These reactions are usually seen in the first 1 to 2 days of treatment, and more commonly occur in younger patients (under 30 years). Dystonic reactions are treated by discontinuing the medication and

with diphenhydramine (one 50 mg dose i.m.). Anti-dopamine receptor effects may elevate prolactin levels and lead to impotence, galactorrhea, and amenorrhea. Extrapyramidal movement disorders and tardive dyskinesia may develop with long-term use. Most side effects reverse with cessation of therapy, but in rare cases tardive dyskinesia persists indefinitely. The risk of permanent tardive dyskinesia is believed to increase with longer duration of treatment and increased cumulative dose. Patients taking metoclopramide should be made aware of this. Unfortunately, given the absence of alternatives, many patients are willing to take the risk.

Domperidone

Domperidone peripherally blocks dopamine receptors (D$_2$). Its effects in the stomach are similar to metoclopramide, and include improved antroduodenal coordination and inhibition of fundic accommodation to promote gastric emptying, with limited effects outside the proximal gastrointestinal tract. Although domperidone does not cross the blood–brain barrier, it does have antiemetic effects through actions on the chemoreceptor

159

trigger zone (outside the blood–brain barrier). It has no prokinetic or antiemetic actions through serotonin-mediated pathways. In studies it has decreased symptoms, reduced hospitalization rates, and improved gastric emptying. Although not FDA approved, it is available outside the US, including Canada and Mexico. Usual doses range from 10 to 30 mg taken four times daily. Side effects are rare and few. Hyperprolactinemia (and its complications) may develop due to minimal blood–brain barrier crossing in the anterior pituitary.

Cisapride

Cisapride has prokinetic effects through serotonin receptor (5-HT$_4$) linked cholinergic stimulation in the myenteric plexus and direct smooth muscle contractility via serotonin receptor (5-HT$_3$) blockade. Serontonin receptor (5-HT$_3$) antagonism may additionally provide for antiemetic activity. Prokinetic effects are not limited to the proximal gastrointestinal tract, and include increased antral, small bowel, and colonic motility. It increases gastric emptying, reduces duodenogastric reflux, and improves antroduodenal coordination. It has been useful for treating gastroparesis due to a variety of underlying etiologies. The usual doses range from 10 to 20 mg taken twice to four times daily.

Cisapride is metabolized by the cytochrome P450 system. Drugs that interact with this system may lead to increased serum levels. High levels of cisapride can prolong the cardiac QT interval, and predispose to life-threatening ventricular arrhythmias, such as torsades de pointes. Drugs that commonly have such interactions, and that should be avoided in the setting of cisapride, include macrolide antibiotics, azole antifungals, and protease inhibitors. Cisapride should be avoided in patients with personal or family history of QT prolongation and in those at increased risk for arrhythmias. Cisapride has

been withdrawn from the market because of reports of the numerous drug interactions that may lead to cardiac arrhythmias, and is only available through limited access protocols directly from the manufacturer under careful FDA scrutiny. The more common side effects of cisapride are related to its physiologic action, and include abdominal cramping and diarrhea.

Bethanecol

Bethanecol is a muscarinic agonist that stimulates gastrointestinal smooth muscle through actions on muscarinic cholinergic receptors. However, this does not occur in a coordinated fashion. Many studies have demonstrated an increase in gastric motor activity, but have failed to show improvement in gastric emptying. It has no known antiemetic effect. The usual dose is 25 mg, four times daily. Common side effects include abdominal cramping, flushing, diaphoresis, salivation, nausea, and vomiting. Rarely, it may cause decreases in blood pressure and atrial fibrillation. Because of its limited efficacy and side effects, bethanecol is rarely used for gastroparesis.

Erythromycin

Erythromycin is a motilin receptor agonist that is believed to stimulate the gastroduodenal migrating motor complex. It is a potent stimulator of gastric emptying, and leads to strong, lumen-obliterating contractions that increase both solid and liquid emptying. Erythromycin has proven useful in diabetic, postsurgical, and scleroderma-associated dysmotility. The usual dosage is much less than that needed for antibiotic use, and starts at 50 mg, four times daily. An available liquid preparation may be better tolerated, and more easily absorbed as compared to the solid form. Common side effects include abdominal cramping and nausea. Its long-term use may be limited because of tachyphylaxis.

Erythromycin is typically used in the short-term setting for acute flares of symptoms.

Antiemetics

Some prokinetic medications have antiemetic properties that control symptoms of nausea and vomiting. However, some patients with gastroparesis have refractory symptoms that require additional control. In this setting a variety of the commonly used antiemetics are acceptable, such as phenothiazine derivatives, provided that side effects are tolerable. In general their long-term use should be avoided if possible, as their anticholinergic effects may actually worsen gastric emptying. However, in patients with severe symptoms they may be used chronically.

Surgical therapy

Patients with severe symptoms that are refractory to dietary and medical therapy may be candidates for surgical treatment. Venting gastrostomy tubes can alleviate symptoms of nausea, vomiting, and bloating. This strategy has enabled patients to gain weight, improve functional status, and may allow for the discontinuation of prokinetic medications. Jejunosotomy tubes can help patients that are unable to maintain adequate hydration and nutrition. Gastrostomy tubes can be placed surgically, endoscopically, or under fluoroscopic guidance. Jejunostomy tubes are usually placed surgically, but have been placed percutaneously under endoscopic guidance. Combined gastrostomy–jejunostomy tube placement can be performed under endoscopic or fluoroscopic guidance through a gastric puncture site.

More radical surgical approaches such as subtotal gastrectomy with Roux-en-Y reconstruction or operative anastomotic revisions should only be entertained after other therapeutic measures have been exhausted. Few reports describe their utility in the management of gastroparesis.

Alternative therapy

Patients with postoperative and idiopathic nausea and vomiting have improved with acupuncture. It should be considered for refractory symptoms of gastroparesis as an adjunct to other measures.

Future therapeutic approaches

Gastric pacing

Gastric pacing involves the surgical placement of electrical pacing wires into the gastric serosa. Theoretically, this technique is useful for gastric dysrhythmias, and works by overriding the intrinsic gastric slow wave activity to normalize gastric rhythms. In initial investigations it has demonstrated varying results in terms of symptom improvement and gastric emptying. Other therapeutic mechanisms of gastric pacing have been proposed, such as centrally mediated effects on nausea and vomiting, and alteration of visceral sensitivity. Currently, gastric pacing is investigational, and limited to specialized centers with expertise in gastrointestinal motility.

Medical therapy

With increased understanding of gastrointestinal motor physiology, we anticipate new medications for gastroparesis. Pharmaceutical innovations will likely occur in the areas of cholinergic stimulants, motilin agonists, opiate antagonists, cholecystokinin antagonists, and selective 5-HT$_4$ agonists.

Further reading

Bityutskiy LP, Soykan I, McCallum RW. Viral gastroparesis – clinical characteristics and long-term outcomes. *Am J Gastroenterol* 1997; 92(9): 1501–1504.

Hasler WL. Disorders of gastric emptying. In Yamada T, Alpers DH (eds) *Textbook of Gastroenterology* 3rd edn, vol. 1, Phildelphia PA: Lippincott Williams & Wilkins; 1999, pp. 1341–1369.

Hornbuckle K, Barnett JL. The diagnosis and work-up of the patient with gastroparesis. *J Clin Gastroenterol* 2000; 30(2): 117–124.

Horowitz M, Fraser RJL. Gastroparesis: diagnosis and management. *Scand J Gastroenterol* 1995; 30: 7–16.

Koch KL. Electrogastrography: physiological basis and clinical application in diabetic gastropathy. *Diabetes Technol Ther* 2001; 3(1): 51–62.

Koch KL. Nausea: an approach to a symptom. *Clin Perspect Gastroenterol* 2001; Sept/Oct: 285–297.

Ladabaum U, Hasler WL. Novel approaches to the treatment of nausea and vomiting. *Dig Dis* 1999; 17(3): 125–132.

Parkman HP, Harris AD, Krevsky B, *et al.* Gastroduodenal motility and dysmotility: an update on techniques available for evaluation. *Am J Gastroenterol* 1995; 90(6): 869–892.

Patterson D, Abell T, Rothstein R, *et al.* A double-blind multicenter comparison of domperidone and metoclopramide in the treatment of diabetic patients with symptoms of gastroparesis. *Am J Gastroenterol* 1999; 94(5): 1230–1234.

Quigley EM. Pharmacotherapy of gastroparesis. *Expert Opin Pharmacother* 2000; 1(5): 881–887.

Rabine JC, Barnett JL. Management of the patient with gastroparesis. *J Clin Gastroenterol* 2001; 32(1): 11–18.

Soykan I, Sivri B, Sarosiek I, *et al.* Demography, clinical characteristics, psychological and abuse profile, treatment, and long-term follow-up of patients with gastroparesis. *Dig Dis Sci* 1998; 43(11): 2398–2404.

Sturm A, Holtman G, Goebell H. Prokinetics in patients with gastroparesis: a systemic analysis. *Digestion* 1999; 60(5): 422–427.

Talley NJ, Verlinden M, Geenen DJ, *et al.* Effects of a motilin receptor agonist (ABT-229) on upper gastrointestinal symptoms in type 1 diabetes mellitus: a randomized, double blind, placebo controlled trial. *Gut* 2001; 49(3): 395–401.

Chapter 11

Non-Ulcer Dyspepsia

David A. Katzka and David C. Metz

CHAPTER OUTLINE

Introduction

Dyspepsia is a non-specific descriptive term generally defined as pain or discomfort centered in the upper abdomen (Box 11.1). To the lay individual dyspepsia is essentially equivalent to "indigestion" though the pain or discomfort may not necessarily be a consequence of dietary indiscretion. Certainly, the vagueness of these terms leads to a host of different symptoms. For example, discomfort may include upper abdominal fullness, early satiety, bloating, or nausea. Similarly, the pain threshold for individual patients will also vary leading certain patients to perceive their symptoms as a "pain" whilst others may only describe "discomfort". As a result, the list of diagnoses ascribed to dyspepsia is long and may include peptic ulcer disease, gastric cancer, reflux disease, gallstones, pancreatic cancer or pancreatitis, and numerous others. In its broadest sense, dyspepsia may be "uninvestigated" or "undifferentiated" (Box 11.1). These all-inclusive terms encompass all patients presenting to physicians with a general complaint of upper abdominal pain or discomfort reflecting disease states that are easily diagnosed with imaging studies (e.g. peptic ulcers, gastric cancer, erosive esophagitis, cholecystitis, or pancreatitis) as well as other less-easily diagnosed conditions in which preliminary imaging studies may be within normal limits (e.g. gastroduodenal dysrhythmias, accommodation abnormalities, dysmotility syndromes, or non-erosive reflux disease). The absence of easily recognizable organic disease has led some authorities to coin the term "functional dyspepsia" for the latter group of conditions all of which have symptoms referable to the upper gastrointestinal tract. While the term "functional dyspepsia" has some utility when it is used to distinguish upper gastrointestinal

Box 11.1 Description of terms

Dyspepsia
   pain or discomfort centered in the upper
   abdomen
Undifferentiated (uninvestigated) dyspepsia
   an all-inclusive term prior to structural
   evaluation
Non-ulcer (functional) dyspepsia
   dyspepsia with a normal structural study
   (endoscopy or barium X-ray)
Ulcer dyspepsia
   dyspepsia in the presence of peptic
   ulceration
Ulcer-like dyspepsia
   ulcer-like pain with a normal structural study
Motility-like dyspepsia
   abdominal discomfort, bloating, fullness,
   or early satiety with a normal structural
   study
Reflux-like dyspepsia
   non-erosive reflux disease presenting with
   epigastric discomfort as the predominant
   symptom

conditions without obvious organic causes from irritable bowel syndrome, which generally refers to functional disease of the lower gastrointestinal tract, it clearly describes a syndrome with many potential causes, at least some of which are explained by organic abnormalities (e.g. gastroparesis). An alternative approach to the subdivision of "undifferentiated" or "uninvestigated" dyspepsia requires a structural examination of the upper gastrointestinal tract (i.e. an upper endoscopy or barium study). Structural evaluation permits a distinction to be made between "ulcer dyspepsia" and "non-ulcer dyspepsia" (Box 11.1). It has clinical utility in that it readily distinguishes the easily diagnosed (and treated) peptic ulcer patient from the less easily diagnosed (and treated) non-ulcer dyspeptic patient. Non-ulcer dyspepsia is thus a syndrome defined by its name: that is, a patient with ulcer-like symptoms but without the finding of an ulcer on radiographic or endoscopic evaluation. Its prevalence is high

(up to 25% of the U.S. population in some surveys). Over the years, physicians have tried to break down this non-specific term into specific subcategories. One of the first attempts was to divide non-ulcer dyspepsia patients into those with ulcer-like, motility-like, or reflux-like symptoms (Box 11.1). With newer and more precise methods of quantifying gastric-acid secretion, motility, and visceral perception and accommodation, non-ulcer dyspepsia now encompasses many different putative pathophysiologic processes with many more emerging as we learn more about the underlying mechanisms. With these recent advances in our understanding of what causes dyspepsia, treatment options have expanded to include a number of new (and some older) classes of drugs in addition to traditional therapies such as acid suppression or prokinetics. In this chapter we will review new insights into the pathophysiology, diagnosis, and management of non-ulcer dyspepsia. Peptic ulcer disease, GERD, gastric cancer, and gastroparesis are discussed elsewhere in this volume and hepatobiliary and pancreatic diseases are discussed in a later volume.

Definition

As in any syndrome, assignment of specific symptoms is often based on arbitrary or anecdotal criteria. As a result, consensus panels of international experts have tried to agree on specific definitions. One such conference put forth the Rome II criteria for non-ulcer (or functional) dyspepsia (Box 11.2), defining it as "at least 12 weeks, which need not be consecutive, in the preceding 12 months of persistent or recurrent dyspepsia (i.e. pain or discomfort centered in the upper abdomen) without evidence of organic disease (including an upper endoscopy) that is likely to explain the symptoms and without evidence that the dyspepsia is exclusively relieved by defecation or associated with the onset of a change in stool frequency or stool form (i.e. not irritable bowel syndrome)."

> **Box 11.2** Rome II criteria for non-ulcer (or functional) dyspepsia
>
> At least 12 weeks, which need not be consecutive, in the preceding 12 months of:
> 1. persistent or recurrent dyspepsia (pain or discomfort centered in the upper abdomen)
> 2. no evidence of organic disease (including an upper endoscopy) that is likely to explain the symptoms
> 3. no evidence that dyspepsia is exclusively relieved by defecation or associated with the onset of a change in stool frequency or stool form (i.e. not irritable bowel syndrome)

> **Box 11.3** Rome II subdivisions for non-ulcer (or functional) dyspepsia
>
> **1. Subgroup B1a**
> ulcer-like dyspepsia in which the predominant (most bothersome) symptom is pain centered in the upper abdomen
>
> **2. Subgroup B1b**
> dysmotility-like dyspepsia in which the predominant symptom is an unpleasant or troublesome non-painful sensation (i.e. a discomfort) centered in the upper abdomen (this sensation may be characterized by, or associated with, upper abdominal fullness, early satiety, bloating, or nausea)
>
> **3. Subgroup B1c**
> unspecified (non-specific) dyspepsia in symptomatic patients whose symptoms do not fulfill the criteria for ulcer-like or dysmotility-like dyspepsia

The Rome II consensus group also attempted to further divide dyspeptic patients into one of three functional subgroups as follows, defining:

1. ulcer-like dispepsia as the predominant (most bothersome) symptom is pain centered in the upper abdomen

2. dysmotility-like dyspepsia in which the predominant symptom is an unpleasant or troublesome non-painful sensation (i.e. a discomfort) centered in the upper abdomen (this sensation may be characterized by or associated with upper abdominal fullness, early satiety, bloating, or nausea), or

3. unspecified (or non-specific) dyspepsia in symptomatic patients whose symptoms do not fulfill the criteria for ulcer-like or dysmotility-like dyspepsia (Box 11.3).

The most recent consensus conference attempted to separate GERD as a truly distinct entity thereby failing to include a reflux-like dyspepsia subgroup.

Although generally helpful, many patients have overlapping symptoms or their symptoms do not fit clearly into a specific category, underscoring how imprecise our understanding of these patients can be. Moreover, studies have shown that symptom complexes alone are unreliable in trying to determine the underlying specific pathophysiology (or therapeutic approach) in these patients. Nevertheless, these definitions are at least worthwhile for initial categorization of dyspeptic patients thereby aiding their early evaluation and treatment.

Pathophysiology

In general, the pathophysiology of non-ulcer dyspepsia (Box 11.4) is separated into three primary categories: acid-peptic disease, abnormal motility, and visceral hyperalgesia. There are two possible explanations for why certain individuals may have the ability to sense acid without having gross evidence of endoscopic or histologic injury. First, some patients with non-ulcer dyspepsia may actually have underlying GERD. These individuals sense abnormal esophageal acid exposure as epigastric pain rather than presenting with the more typical substernal burning pain characterized as heartburn. Indeed, prolonged

Box 11.4 Pathophysiology of non-ulcer dyspepsia

1. Acid-peptic disease
   i) undiagnosed non-erosive reflux disease
   ii) prolonged duodenal acid exposure

2. Abnormal gastroduodenal motility
   i) defective fundal relaxation (poor gastric compliance)
   ii) gastric dysrhythmias (bradygastria or tachygastria)
   iii) primary muscular defects (ineffective or uncoordinated contractions)
       neuropathic
       post-infectious

3. Visceral hyperalgesia
   i) hypersensitivity to normal stimuli
       defective mechanoreceptors
       defective chemoreceptors
   ii) excessive sensitivity to subclinical pathologic stimuli
       defective mechanoreceptors
       defective chemoreceptors
   iii) post-infectious
   iv) psychogenic factors

4. *Helicobacter pylori* gastritis

Abnormal gastroduodenal motility in non-ulcer dyspepsia was first described in patients who exhibited a delay in gastric emptying as determined on solid-phase gastric emptying scanning (i.e. gastroparesis of varying severity). Typically, after ingesting a standardized meal containing technetium labeled egg whites these patients demonstrate significantly longer retention of radioactivity in the stomach as compared with normal subjects (see Chapter 10). Within the past decade through the use of more sophisticated physiologic testing methodologies evaluating different aspects of gastric motility, other putative disorders have been described. Such potential abnormalities include defective gastric fundal relaxation where poor gastric compliance causes the gastric wall to lose its ability to stretch and accommodate an ingested meal. Defects of gastric compliance can be demonstrated through barostat studies, which permit assessment of gastric wall tension under various conditions. Gastric dysrhythmias have also been demonstrated in certain non-ulcer dyspepsia patients. Under normal fasting conditions the gastric pacemaker located on the greater curvature of the distal gastric corpus fires three times per minute. Instead, in a dysrhythmia the pacemaker may fire too slowly (i.e. bradygastria) or too rapidly (i.e. tachygastria). Such abnormalities may lead to defective coupling of the electrical stimulus for muscular contraction with the actual muscular response. Gastric rhythms can be demonstrated with electrogastrography in which cutaneous electrodes are placed on the anterior abdominal wall to detect electric impulses generated by the enteric nervous system. Primary muscular defects have also been proposed in certain non-ulcer dyspepsia patients. These include low-amplitude (i.e. ineffective) contractions as well as antropyloroduodenal motility patterns that lack appropriate coordination. Although certain systemic disease states such as diabetes mellitus, or collagen vascular diseases such as scleroderma, are well known

ambulatory pH monitoring in such patients may reveal a close correlation between the onset of epigastric pain or discomfort and the presence of acid refluxate in the distal esophagus. It is unclear at this time whether the dyspepsia in these individuals is a consequence of pain that is referred from the esophagus to the epigastrium, or whether there is an increased sensitivity to acid in the proximal stomach (i.e. the cardia). A second possible acid-peptic explanation for dyspepsia was recently suggested by investigators who demonstrated that patients with non–ulcer dyspepsia might have prolonged duodenal acid exposure as a consequence of abnormal gastroduodenal motility leading to pooling and prolonged unbuffered duodenal exposure to gastric acid.

to be associated with gastric dysmotility, most non-ulcer dyspepsia patients do not have obvious underlying organic causes for their dysmotility. Some authorities have suggested that gastroduodenal dysmotility in such individuals may be a consequence of prior viral infection, but definitive proof of this hypothesis is lacking. Other authorities have suggested that subclinical autonomic or vagal neuropathy may be responsible for the dysmotility in certain non-ulcer dyspepsia patients. In general these dysmotility syndromes are currently regarded as idiopathic and the precise roles they may play in the generation of dyspepsia remains hypothetical.

The concept of gastroduodenal hyperalgesia implies hypersensitivity of these organs to various stimuli. Specifically, normal (i.e. physiologic) stimuli may be sensed in these individuals in contrast to normal individuals who lack this ability. Alternatively, subclinical pathophysiologic stimuli that may usually be perceived as subtle or non-bothersome by normal subjects may be felt as pain or discomfort by certain non-ulcer dyspepsia patients. Barostat studies have demonstrated a leftwards shift of gastric sensory thresholds to graded balloon distension in certain non-ulcer dyspepsia patients suggesting a muscular mechanoreceptor defect. However, defective mucosal chemoreceptor function may also play a role. Thus, gastroduodenal hyperalgesia may be the final common pathway to explain both acid-peptic-type symptoms as well as dysmotility-type symptoms. Post-viral etiologies have also been proposed as the underlying cause for the hypersensitivity hypothesis. It should be noted that a similar mechanism has also been proposed to explain the development of irritable bowel syndrome. Others have suggested that pyschogenic factors may also be important in the generation of gastroduodenal hypersensitivity. Indeed, numerous studies have demonstrated that patients with non-ulcer dyspepsia may have a higher prevalence of psychiatric disorders and experimentally evoked stresses may lower sensory thresholds in the gastrointestinal tract. The potential for underlying psychiatric abnormalities may be important when deciding upon possible treatment strategies for non-ulcer dyspepsia.

Finally, the potential role of *Helicobacter pylori* infection in the development of non-ulcer dyspepsia has been hotly debated in the literature. Since *H. pylori* gastritis clearly is a pathologic state, it is tempting to speculate that gastritis alone may lead to dyspepsia, even in the absence of documented ulcer disease. However, controlled studies have failed to consistently demonstrate improvement in symptoms after eradication of the infection. It may well be that there is a small subset of non-ulcer dyspepsia patients in whom *H. pylori* gastritis is causative (perhaps 20%) but, to date, investigators have been unable to identify criteria that will predict which patients will respond. It has also been proposed that *H. pylori* gastritis may lead to irreversible damage that cannot always be reversed by curing the infection although it must be stressed that the vast majority of infected individuals do not have dyspepsia at all. *H.pylori* gastritis is discussed in more detail in Chapter 8.

Diagnosis

The specific criteria for diagnosing non-ulcer dyspepsia have been reviewed in the preceding sections. Despite the pitfalls in attempting to subdivide non-ulcer dyspepsia according to the predominant presenting symptoms, some investigators have attempted to subclassify non-ulcer dyspepsia further. Acid-peptic non-ulcer dyspepsia presents with an epigastric burning sensation, typically relieved by food ingestion. Patients with gastroparesis describe early satiety, and pain or discomfort which presents after eating. Those with poor gastric compliance may also describe early satiety and pain or discomfort after ingestion.

As is implied by the term non-ulcer dyspepsia, the cornerstone of initial diagnostic testing is an upper endoscopy (i.e. non-ulcer dyspepsia is by definition a diagnosis of exclusion). Endoscopy rules out peptic ulcer disease, erosive esophagitis, or other inflammatory or neoplastic diseases of the upper gastrointestinal tract. However, it is controversial whether all undifferentiated dyspeptics require endoscopy. For example, certain authorities maintain that for young, seemingly healthy individuals with chronic intermittent dyspeptic symptoms, but without "alarm" symptoms for underlying serious organic disease such as dysphagia, bleeding, vomiting, anemia or weight loss, the most cost-effective approach to management may actually be an empiric trial of acid suppression instead. On the other hand there also are data suggesting that early endoscopy may be particularly useful even in young patients without alarm symptoms because it provides reassurance which has a positive effect on symptoms. The threshold for performing an early upper endoscopy is much lower in older patients (e.g. those over the age of 45 years or so) because the likelihood of finding serious underlying organic pathology rises. We generally follow the American Gastroenterological Association guidelines, which recommend diagnostic testing for *Helicobacter pylori* infection (i.e. a serum antibody or urea breath test) followed by a 4 to 6 week empiric trial of acid suppression (if negative) or eradication antibiotics (if positive) in young patients, especially those with acid-peptic-type symptoms. If symptoms persist or recur we then proceed to upper endoscopy. We have a low threshold for performing early endoscopy in older patients and always endoscope patients with alarm symptoms.

Once non-ulcer dyspepsia has been confirmed (i.e. once a normal upper endoscopy has been documented), further evaluation should depend on the predominant symptom complex (i.e. acid–peptic dyspepsia versus motility/hyperalgesia dyspepsia) and the availability of specialized tests. For patients with persistent acid–peptic symptoms, we advocate the use of prolonged ambulatory pH monitoring to evaluate for GERD as an alternative explanation for symptoms. However, not all physicians have pH monitoring readily available. Therefore, treatment with the lowest effective dose of maintenance proton pump inhibitor therapy is a reasonable approach as well. Studies in reflux patients have shown that the diagnostic accuracy of empiric antisecretory therapy approaches that of prolonged ambulatory pHmetry. For patients with motility-type symptoms, we advocate additional testing to at least include a nuclear gastric emptying scan. We generally advocate additional testing (over empiric therapy for gastroparesis) because the available prokinetic medications either have a relatively high incidence of side effects (metoclopramide), are only available on a compassionate use limited investigational new drug (IND) under careful FDA monitoring (cisapride) or are less effective or subject to tachyphylaxis (erythromycin). Domperidone is not available for use in the US because the studies submitted for FDA approval failed to convincingly demonstrate clear correlation between its prokinetic effects and symptom responses. Moreover, as will be discussed later (see p. 171), medications used to treat other dysmotility disorders (i.e. abnormalities of gastric compliance or visceral hyperalgesia) run the risk of slowing gastric emptying further so that they are relatively contraindicated in patients with documented gastroparesis.

If the gastric emptying scan is normal, empiric therapy for the other putative disorders associated with non-ulcer dyspepsia may be tried next. This is because barostat and electrogastrography testing are not generally available. Moreover, while electrogastrography is an essentially painless procedure, barostat testing is cumbersome and uncomfortable requiring transnasal passage of a rather large catheter and also requires a high level of expertise on the part of the testing physician. The water load test has been advocated by some as an alternative method to evaluate gastric compliance but it has not yet gained general acceptance.

As mentioned above (p. 167), the role of *H. pylori* testing in non-ulcer dyspepsia patients is controversial. The general rule of thumb is not to test unless the physician has decided up front that a positive test will lead to active therapy and the response to therapy in non-ulcer dyspepsia patients is poor. It is also important to remember that in areas with low *H. pylori* prevalence, antibody testing has a low positive predictive value. In addition, active testing with invasive (i.e. endoscopic biopsy) and non-invasive methods (i.e. breath test or stool test) is subject to false-negative results in the presence of proton pump inhibitor therapy. Figure 11.1 illustrates our general approach to patients suspected of having non-ulcer dyspepsia.

Treatment (Box 11.5)

General measures

Reassurance is a very important part of therapy for patients with non-ulcer dyspepsia. Part of this is realistically based in that only a very small minority of patients go on to develop more serious disease states (i.e. frank peptic ulcer disease or severe gastroparesis) on follow-up studies. Second, the high placebo response rate usually seen in these patients reinforces the important role of psychological factors in mediating these symptoms. The role of dietary manipulation is unclear. For some patients, spicy food precipitates dyspepsia whereas for patients with the reflux equivalent of non-ulcer dyspepsia avoidance of high-volume high-fat meals, alcohol, chocolate, raw onions, and other foods known to precipitate reflux disease may be useful. For patients with delayed gastric emptying high-fat and high-fiber foods are the most problematic. Frequent snacking rather than regular ingestion of large meals is also beneficial in some individuals.

Medications

For acid-peptic-type non-ulcer dyspepsia, antisecretory therapy is generally useful. While histamine H_2-receptor antagonists may be effective in some individuals these agents are often limited by the need for twice daily therapy. We generally advocate once daily proton pump inhibitors instead. For best effects, proton pump inhibitors should be taken 30 to 60 minutes before breakfast. It is important that patients do not take these medications on an empty stomach as their efficacy is reduced. If there is no or incomplete control of symptoms, the dosage may be increased to twice daily (with the second dose being administered before dinner), but if symptoms still persist antisecretory therapy can be deemed to have failed at this stage and alternative therapies should be sought. The appropriate duration of antisecretory therapy for acid-peptic non-ulcer dyspepsia is controversial but we prefer not to treat for longer than 2 months without reassessing the patient carefully. In contrast to GERD in which long-term maintenance therapy is required, non-ulcer dyspepsia is a condition that tends to wax and wane such that intermittent courses of therapy are required during symptomatic periods, but drug holidays can be used during the intervening periods when the patient is feeling well. We feel strongly that the lowest effective dose of therapy be used to limit activation of the gastric-acid secretory feedback loop which leads to hypergastrinemia and ECL-cell hyperplasia with the potential for rebound

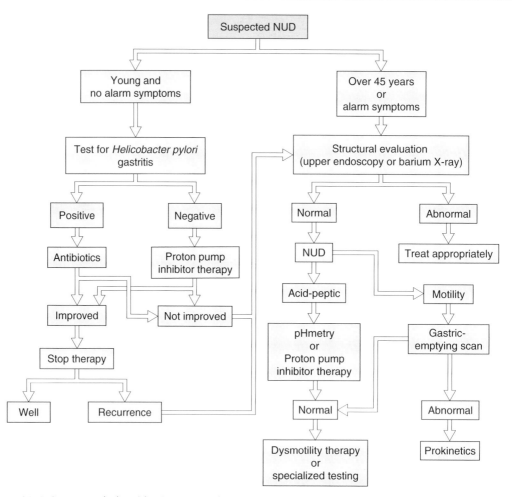

Figure 11.1 Suggested algorithmic approach to patients with suspected non-ulcer dyspepsia (NUD).

hypersecretion after drug withdrawal. Therapy for documented gastroparesis is discussed in depth elsewhere in this volume (see Chapter 10).

Occasionally non-ulcer dyspepsia patients with symptoms suggestive of gastroparesis but normal gastric emptying respond well to prokinetic therapy. In these patients we generally advocate starting with 10 mg of the dopamine agonist, metoclopramide, 30 to 60 minutes before meals with an increase of up to 20 mg four times daily if needed. Side effects are unfortunately common with metoclopramide including agitation, galactorrhea, restlessness, and acute dystonia. Concerning long-term side effects include irreversible tar-

dive dyskinesia and gynecomastia. As a result, it is important for physicians to severely caution patients about these effects. Some physicians ask their patients to sign consent forms which describe these warnings. The motilin agonist, erythromycin, has limited efficacy and is used only occasionally in our practice. Cisapride was withdrawn from the general US market because of reports of torsades des pointes and sudden death due to QT prolongation (especially when used in conjunction with other agents that have similar effects). This agent is available under a limited IND through the manufacturer under careful FDA scrutiny, which requires objective documentation of need (e.g. prolonged gastric empty-

Box 11.5 Treatment of non-ulcer dyspepsia

1. General measures
  i) reassurance
  ii) dietary manipulation

2. Medications
  i) antisecretory therapy
    histamine H$_2$-receptor antagonists
    proton pump inhibitors
  ii) prokinetics
    metoclopramide
    erythromycin
    cisapride
    domperidone
    tegaserod
  iii) gastric compliance enhancers
    anticholinergics
    clonidine
    sumitriptan
  iv) visceral perception blockers
    imipramine
    selective serotonin receptor antagonists

3. Psychologic therapy
  i) stress reduction
    exercise
    acupuncture
    formal courses
    psychiatric medications
  ii) specific therapies
    biofeedback
    hypnosis
    talk therapy (behavioral or psychotherapy)

cussed above (see p. 168), domperidone is not available in the US. Dosages are similar to those for metoclopramide.

Tegaserod, a new 5-HT$_3$ agonist, is already available in Canada and Europe and will likely be released soon in the US for patients with constipation-predominant irritable bowel syndrome. Tegaserod has potential use for patients with gastroparesis but it has not been well studied yet for this indication.

We have a hierarchical approach to patients with suspected or documented gastric compliance abnormalities starting with anticholinergics and progressing to clonidine and sumitriptan. Specifically, we generally start with sublingual hyocyamine 0.125 mg taken before meals, though many other anticholinergics may be useful. Some individuals appear to prefer longer acting anticholinergics such as hyoscyamine prescribed twice daily. If these fail, then clonidine 0.1 mg taken 30 minutes before the meal is used. In some patients, sumitriptan 12.5 to 25 mg before the meal can be used. All these medications have potential side effects (anticholinergics: dry mouth, fatigue; clonidine: hypotension, headache; sumitriptan: myocardial and intestinal ischemia) so that the physician has to monitor patients carefully.

Finally, low-dose tricyclic antidepressants such as imipramine are very effective for suspected gastroduodenal hyperalgesia in our experience. It is important to emphasize that much lower doses should be used for this indication than are usually employed for depression. In our experience many patients need as little as 10 to 20 mg nightly. Higher doses may, in fact, lead to inhibition of gastric emptying and may make symptoms worse. Some physicians use selective serotonin receptor antagonists instead of tricyclic antidepressants because of their inhibition of serotonin, a peptide known to be very important in mediating gastrointestinal afferent sensation. Again, low doses of these agents may be very effective.

ing). This is a rather time-consuming and cumbersome process so that many physicians have elected not to seek IND approval for their patients. In our experience, cisapride has been very helpful for certain eligible patients. The usual dose is 10 to 20 mg taken 30 to 60 minutes before meals and at bedtime. Domperidone is an attractive alternative prokinetic as it has peripheral actions similar to metoclopramide without central nervous system effects because it tends not to cross the blood–brain barrier. Unfortunately, as dis-

Psychologic therapy

Because stress, anxiety, and somatosization may be part of the etiology of non-ulcer dyspepsia, psychological approaches should be considered in select individuals. Generalized therapy for stress reduction may include exercise, acupuncture, formal stress-reduction courses, and medication. More specific therapies such as biofeedback, hypnosis, or talk therapy may be considered. There are some trials demonstrating the benefit of both cognitive behavioral therapy and psychotherapy over no treatment. Which specific treatment is most beneficial is unclear and most likely patient dependent. The role of anxiolytics and antidepressants (other than those mentioned) is unclear as a primary therapy but may be useful if concordant psychiatric disease is present. As mentioned previously, the beneficial effects of some psychiatric medications on visceral hyperalgesia is generally accepted.

Conclusions

Non-ulcer or functional dyspepsia is defined by a symptom complex but represents a heterogeneous group of disorders. Possible etiologies include acid hypersensitivity, gastroduodenal hyperalgesia, and various forms of dysmotility. The therapies are protean including motility agents, acid suppression, and visceral pain reducers, as well as non-pharmacologic approaches. A basic evaluation including endoscopy and gastric emptying scans (and sometimes prolonged ambulatory pH studies) are usually required with much of the treatment initiated empirically because of lack of availability or documented utility for some of the more sophisticated testing methods required for definitive diagnosis.

Further reading

Bytzer P, Schaffalitzky de Muckadell OB. Prediction of major pathologic conditions in dyspeptic patients referred for endoscopy. A prospective validation study of a scoring system. *Scand J Gastroenterol* 1992; 27(11): 987–992.

Chen JDZ, Schirmer BD, McCallum RW. Serosal and cutaneous recordings of gastric myoelectric activity in patients with gastroparesis. *Am J Physiol* 1994; 266: G90–G98.

Distrutti E, Azpiroz F, Soldevilla A, Malagelade J-R. Gastric wall tension determines perception of gastric distention. *Gastroenterology* 1999; 116: 1035–1042.

Drossman DA (ed) *The Functional Gastrointestinal Disorders* 2nd edn. Mclean VA: Degnon Associates; 2000.

Sansom M, Verhagen AMT, VanBerge Henegouwen GP, Smout AJPM. Abnormal clearance of exogenous acid and increased acid sensitivity of the proximal duodenum in dyspeptic patients. *Gastroenterology* 1999; 116: 515–520.

Schmulson MJ, Mayer EA. Evolving concepts in irritable bowel syndrome. *Curr Opin Gastroenterol* 1999; 15: 16–21.

Tack J, Piessevaux H, Coulie B, Caenepeel P, Janssens J. Role of impaired gastric accomodation to a meal in functional dyspepsia. *Gastroenterology* 1998; 115: 1346–1352.

Talley NJ, Silverstein MD, Agreus L, Nyren O, Sonnenberg A, Holtmann G. **AGA** technical review: evaluation of dyspepsia. *Gastroenterology* 1998; 114(3): 582–595.

Talley NJ, Vakil N, Ballard ED II, Fennerty MB. Absence of benefit of eradicating Helicobacter pylori in patients with nonulcer dyspepsia. *New Engl J Med* 1999; 341: 1106–1111.

Thumshirn M, Camilleri M, Choi M-G, Zinsmeister AR. Modulation of gastric sensory and motor functions by nitrergic and alpha-2 adrenergic agents in humans. *Gastroenterology* 1999; 116: 573–585.

Foreign Bodies of the Upper Gastrointestinal Tract

Michelle Beilstein and David A. Katzka

CHAPTER OUTLINE

Introduction

In the US, it is estimated that 1500 people die annually of ingested foreign bodies of the upper gastrointestinal tract. The highest incidence, up to 80% of foreign body ingestions, occurs in children aged 6 months to 3 years, followed by edentulous adults, prisoners, psychiatric patients, and individuals impaired by alcohol ingestion. Dentures are the most common risk factor associated with esophageal foreign bodies in adults, secondary to compromise of tactile sensitivity of the palate. Commonly ingested foreign bodies in children, adults, psychiatric patients, or prisoners are listed in Table 12.1. In the psychiatric population often many objects are involved and recurrence rates range from 2.7% to 10%.

Pathophysiology

The esophagus is susceptible to foreign-body impaction because of four normal physiological narrowings including

- 15 cm from the incisors at the cricopharyengeal muscle or upper esophageal sphincter
- 23 cm from the incisors at the level of the aortic arch
- 27 cm from the incisors at the level of the left main stem bronchus
- 40 cm from the incisors at the level of the diaphragmatic hiatus or gastroesophageal junction.

Abnormalities of the esophagus also predispose patients to foreign body impaction. Such abnormalities are listed in Box 12.1 and include: peptic strictures, Schatzki's rings, esophageal webs, esophageal cancer, achalasia,

Table 12.1 Commonly ingested foreign bodies

Children	Adults
coins	meat
bones	bones
pins	pills
jacks	coins
batteries	dental hardware
marbles	toothpicks

Prisoners and psychiatric patients
toothbrushes
silverware
batteries
razorblades

Box 12.1 Common causes of foreign-body obstruction

Normal physiological narrowings of the esophagus
upper esophageal sphincter
aortic arch
left main-stem bronchus
diaphragmatic hiatus

Abnormal narrowings of the esophagus
peptic strictures
Schatzki's ring
esophageal webs
esophageal cancer
achalasia
diffuse esophageal spasm
scleroderma
myasthenia gravis
myotonic dystrophies
intrathoracic masses
congestive heart failure with an enlarged left atrium

diffuse esophageal spasm, as well as dysfunctional esophageal motility from such diseases as scleroderma, myasthenia gravis and muscular dystrophies. Abnormalities in the thorax such as intrathoracic masses or congestive heart failure with an enlarged left atrium also lead to narrowing of the esophagus leaving it prone to foreign-body impaction.

Most foreign objects that pass through the esophagus and into the stomach will pass spontaneously, but certain objects can have difficulty navigating the pylorus and the duodenal sweep. Of note, objects wider than 2 cm and longer than 5 cm tend to lodge in the stomach unable to pass though the pylorus, and objects longer than 10 cm tend to hang up in the duodenal sweep and can lead to perforation.

Diagnosis

Diagnosis is based on a careful patient history, history from an observer, physical examination, and radiographs. A summary is provided in Table 12.2.

History

The patient may be able to identify what was swallowed, but patient localization of the level of impaction is unreliable. One study reveals that 93% of patients with esophageal foreign bodies felt symptoms immediately after swallowing the foreign body. Interestingly, in up to 50% of patients who complain of a foreign-body sensation no foreign body will be found at endoscopy. In patients with previous gastroesophageal complaints the likelihood of finding a foreign body on endoscopy is increased.

In other instances the patient does not remember the ingestion and presents with symptoms of chest pain, dysphagia, odynophagia, a foreign-body sensation in their esophagus, or drooling with inability to tolerate their secretions. Because of easily compressible, soft tracheal rings children may

Table 12.2 Diagnosis	
Detailed history	often from bystanders
Symptoms	chest pain, dysphagia, odynophagia, drooling, foreign body sensation, *don't forget* respiratory symptoms
Physical examination	assess airway for patency
	signs and symptoms of perforation, crepitus, swelling of the neck, peritonitis or mediastinitis
	signs and symptoms of luminal obstruction, tympanic abdomen, decreased bowel sounds, nausea, or vomiting
Radiographs	Anterior–posterior and lateral neck and chest radiographs, "mouth to anus" in children

also present with respiratory distress when foreign objects are lodged in the proximal esophagus. Symptoms may include cough, stridor, wheezing, apnea, and pneumonia. The longer the foreign object has been in the esophagus the greater the incidence of respiratory symptoms in children. In the mentally ill or small children who do not remember or who cannot tell that they have swallowed an object the presenting symptoms may be choking or the refusal to eat. Thus, a high index of suspicion must be maintained in younger children. A "café coronary" syndrome can occur in adults who have a meat bolus impaction at or just below the cricopharyngeus leading to tracheal compression and resultant respiratory obstruction.

tis; as well as signs of luminal obstruction including tympanic abdomen with decreased bowel sounds, nausea, and vomiting. Pneumonia secondary to aspiration can also occur in these patients. Vascular complications can occur rarely. Usually there is a latency period of 1 to 3 months from the time of foreign-body ingestion to the onset of hemorrhage. Removal of a foreign body is no guarantee that a vascular fistula will not form. Aortoenteric fistulas are most common, but fistulas between the esophagus and carotid or subclavian arteries have also been reported. A patient with a history of foreign-body ingestion and gastrointestinal bleeding should undergo urgent surgical evaluation as surgery is the definitive therapy.

Physical examination

On physical examination airway patency should be assessed and maintained. Perforation and bowel obstruction are complications of foreign-body ingestions that are treated with urgent surgery which should not be delayed by endoscopic evaluation. Thus, it is imperative to look for evidence of perforation on physical examination including erythema, crepitus or swelling of the neck region, and signs of peritonitis or mediastini-

Radiology

Anterior–posterior and lateral radiographs must be obtained of the neck and chest in all patients suspected of foreign-object ingestion. Children should have "mouth-to-anus" screening films when ingestion of a foreign body is suspected. Some objects are radiopaque and can be identified by routine radiographs while others are radiolucent and most likely will not be seen on radiographs (Table 12.3). Radiographs should also always

Table 12.3 Radiopaque versus radiolucent objects

Radiopaque	Radiolucent
coins	thin metal objects
metal buttons	glass
button batteries	wood
safety pins	aluminum
clam shells	plastic
large chicken bones	small fish and chicken bones
narcotic packets	fish cartilage
cocaine packets	peanuts, sunflower seeds, popcorn

be evaluated for signs of perforation – air in the subcutaneous tissue, mediastinum, or beneath the diaphragm. Contrast studies with barium or gastrograffin should not routinely be obtained. Barium coats the esophagus and foreign body obscuring endoscopic visualization. Gastrograffin is contraindicated because if aspirated into the lungs it can lead to a severe chemical pneumonitis.

Management

General management

Eighty to ninety per cent of foreign bodies that reach the gastrointestinal tract will pass spontaneously, but 10% to 20% will require medical and endoscopic intervention and fewer than 1% will require surgery. Most foreign bodies requiring intervention are lodged in the esophagus.

Most foreign objects in the esophagus and stomach can be removed by endoscopy. These patients should remain nothing by mouth until definitive therapy is undertaken. An initial trial of glucagon in a patient with food lodged at the LES to attempt to relax the smooth muscle of the LES and allow for pas-

sage of the object into the stomach can be tried. The literature reports success rates of glucagon to be 12% to 50%. The dose of glucagon is usually 1 to 2 mg i.v. in adults and 0.02 to 0.03 mg/kg, with a maximum dose of 0.5 mg, in children. It is reasonable to repeat the dose after 20 minutes, but if the first two doses are ineffective, further doses are not indicated. Glucagon may precipitate nausea and vomiting and should be used cautiously in patients with insulinomas, pheochromocytomas, or Zollinger–Ellison syndrome. In patients with insulinomas, glucagon may cause the tumor to secrete insulin leading to hypoglycemia requiring therapy with intravenous dextrose. In patients with pheochromocytoma glucagon may cause the tumor to secrete catecholamines leading to severe hypertension which is best treated with phentolamine. Glucagon is unlikely to be successful in patients with esophageal pathology such as peptic strictures, Schatzki's rings, or esophageal carcinoma. The patient may report relief of their discomfort if glucagon is successful in relieving the obstruction. Follow-up films to confirm passage of the foreign body from the esophagus to stomach are necessary. Follow-up endoscopy is warranted to evaluate the esophagus for underlying pathology.

Patients with obstructions from sharp objects, disk batteries lodged in the esophagus, and high-grade obstructions from food impactions, with an inability to manage their secretions require urgent endoscopic intervention. All foreign bodies or food-bolus impactions should be removed from the esophagus once the patient is stabilized. Delayed removal of food-bolus impactions allows the food bolus to soften making extraction more difficult. Delayed removal of food bolus impactions and foreign bodies also increases the risk of perforation secondary to pressure necrosis or direct puncture. In cases where patients are unable to tolerate their secretions, aspiration leading to pneumonia may also occur.

Esophageal foreign objects can be removed via rigid esophagoscopy or flexible endoscopy. Rigid esophagoscopy is most frequently used to remove foreign bodies at the level of the hypopharynx or cricopharyngeus muscle and is only performed under general anesthesia. Flexible endoscopy is the preferred instrument for most foreign bodies at the level of the esophagus, stomach, and duodenum and may be performed under general anesthesia or conscious sedation. Most importantly, special care should be taken to maintain a patent airway at all times and this may require endotracheal intubation especially if the patient has respiratory compromise or has copious secretions that cannot be managed when the patient is sedated. Intubation may also be necessary if the patient is combative or intoxicated, mentally retarded, elderly, or a young child.

The use of an overtube is essential to avoid inadvertently dropping the foreign object into the respiratory tree and allows for safe passage of the endoscope multiple times to retrieve the object if needed. Overtubes also protect the mucosa of the esophagus or stomach from sharp edges of the foreign body or bone fragments in a food-bolus impaction. The risks to passing an overtube which should be included in informed consent include: pharyngeal perforation, esophageal perforation, esophageal tears and lacerations, bleeding from esophageal varices, and gastric mucosal abrasions.

It is often helpful for the endoscopist or surgeon to undergo a "dry run" simulating grasping of a similar object with the equipment intended for use. Equipment needed for endoscopic removal of foreign objects or food-bolus impactions are listed in Box 12.2. One study revealed that the Roth net is best for retrieving smooth objects such as button batteries, and the snare or forceps were best for the removal of sharp objects. They also showed that more experienced endoscopists had higher success rates and faster retrieval times.

Magnetic removal and Foley catheter extraction have been described in the litera-ture. These techniques are not advocated by the authors as they may lead to inadvertently dropping the foreign body into the hypopharynx leading to pulmonary aspiration. In addition, the operators may miss underlying esophageal pathology and may leave radiolucent parts of an esophageal foreign-body behind.

Specific management for different types of foreign objects

See Tables 12.1 and 12.3 for a list of different types of foreign objects.

Food bolus impaction

Meat impaction in the upper and lower esophagus is the most common foreign body in adults. Up to 82% of patients presenting with food-bolus impaction have underlying esophageal pathology; a Schatzki's ring, peptic strictures, achalasia, esophageal webs, or esophageal cancer. Children are rarely affected unless they have congenital defects of the esophagus.

Food bolus impactions particularly predispose to complete esophageal obstruction manifested by salivation and an inability to tolerate secretions. As a result, these patients require urgent endoscopy with airway protection to relieve the obstruction. Once again, all food-bolus impactions should be removed as

---

Box 12.2 Equipment needed for flexible endoscopic esophageal foreign-body disimpaction

Roth net
Rat tooth forceps
Alligator forceps
Polypectomy snare
Polyp grabber
Dormia basket
Overtubes in esophageal and gastric lengths

soon as possible. A trial of glucagon can be given while arrangements are being made for endoscopy, but even if the bolus passes from the esophagus to the stomach endoscopy is required to assess underlying pathology. Most food-bolus impactions can be removed through flexible endoscopy with the use of rat-tooth or alligator forceps, snares, and polyp graspers. Once again, the use of an overtube with this technique is important to protect the airway as multiple passes with the flexible endoscope may be necessary to completely remove the food bolus.

A lot of controversy surrounds the issue of removing the food bolus or passing it into the stomach allowing it to pass naturally. Recently a retrospective study was published evaluating the safety and efficacy of a push technique in treating esophageal food impaction. The push technique is the application of gentle pressure on the esophageal food bolus with the tip of the endoscope after air insufflations of the esophagus. This technique was successful in 97% of patients with no major complications (perforation, aspiration, or bleeding) occurring in any of the 189 patients studied. Thus, it is reasonable to attempt to push the food bolus from the esophagus into the stomach with gentle pressure. If this is unsuccessful extraction via flexible endoscopy with an overtube should be undertaken.

This same group and others have evaluated the safety and efficacy of esophageal dilation for patients with underlying esophageal pathology (peptic strictures, Schatzki's ring, esophageal cancer) directly following foreign-body removal. In this subgroup of 42 patients no complications were noted. Another group performed immediate dilation on 172 patients with no major complications. Thus, in patients with underlying esophageal stricture, dilation immediately following relief of a food-bolus impaction should be considered if the esophageal mucosa is not ulcerated and the procedure is being undertaken in a controlled setting such as an endoscopy unit.

Papain, a meat tenderizer, should not be used because it is associated with hypernatremia, erosion, and esophageal perforation as the tenderizer also tenderizes the mucosa of the esophagus. Coca-Cola and other substances known as fizzies have also been evaluated in the management of esophageal food-bolus impaction. These gas-forming agents distend the esophagus and increase intraluminal pressure above the bolus with the hope of forcing the bolus through the LES (especially when given with glucagon which relaxes the LES). Although they have been effective in small studies, reports of perforation and difficult endoscopic extraction due to further impaction of the bolus make these agents unattractive forms of therapy.

Coins and buttons Small coins such as dimes and pennies, or small buttons rarely cause obstruction when swallowed except in small children, but larger coins, such as quarters, or buttons may impact and obstruct the gastrointestinal lumen. Usually larger coins or buttons will lodge at the level of the cricopharyngeus muscle or just distal to it. Radiographs (anterior–posterior and lateral) of the neck and chest should always be taken in these patients. Even if the child has no complaints, radiographs should be obtained after ingestion as impaction of the esophagus may be asymptomatic in up to 16% of patients. Coins and buttons are usually oriented in the sagittal plane if they are in the trachea and in the frontal plane if they are in the esophagus. Coins or buttons lodged in the esophagus should undergo extraction as soon as possible to avoid complications of fistulas (i.e. aortoenteric or tracheo-esophageal) and perforation.

Endoscopic removal of coins or buttons lodged in the esophagus is the preferred mode of extraction. As with other foreign objects, it is imperative to maintain an airway at all times; this may require endotracheal anesthesia especially in small children. Coins and buttons are most easily removed with either a polypectomy snare, Roth retrieval net, or rat-tooth or alligator forceps. The patient can be placed in the Trendelenberg position to help decrease the risk of dropping the coin or button into the trachea. If the coin or button is small, it can be gently pushed into the stomach and retrieved there, or allowed to pass on its own. Once coins or buttons reach the stomach, they will usually pass without complications. One can allow up to 4 weeks for a coin or button to pass before endoscopically removing it from the stomach. In children and infants who have had prior gastric outlet surgery, the coin or button should be removed endoscopically from the stomach as they probably will not pass on their own. Once past the stomach, surgical removal of objects that remain in the same location for more than 1 week should be considered.

Retrieval of coins or buttons via a Foley-catheter technique or via magnets has been reported. These techniques should be avoided because they may increase the risk of foreign-body aspiration during removal. One small prospective, double-blind, placebo-controlled trial revealed glucagon was less effective than placebo in the dislodgement of esophageal coins in children.

Button batteries In children less than 5 years of age the most commonly ingested battery is the button battery. Button batteries are found in hearing aids, calculators, watches, and small clocks. Battery ingestion can cause injury to the gastrointestinal mucosa in three ways:
- low-voltage burns
- pressure necrosis
- direct corrosive action resulting from an alkaline electrolyte solution released from the battery that is strong enough to cause rapid liquefactive necrosis of tissue.

Radiographs can distinguish between coins and button batteries. Button batteries have a double-density shadow (halo) due to the bi-laminar structure of the battery.

All batteries should be removed endoscopically if possible. The endoscopic removal of button batteries is dependent on the location of the battery and its size. In the esophagus, button batteries should be removed urgently as the alkaline substance acts rapidly on the esophageal mucosa and can lead to esophago-tracheal and esophago-aortic fistulization in a relatively short period of time. Endotracheal anesthesia is required in most patients to protect the airway at all times to avoid dropping the button battery into the trachea where it can lodge in bronchi. Often the battery is pushed into the stomach and retrieved with a Roth retrieval net or basket as biopsy forceps, graspers, and snares are generally not effective.

Once the battery is removed, the involved esophagus must be examined closely by endoscopy to assess the amount of tissue damage. The patient should be placed on antibiotics if significant tissue damage is noted. A barium swallow should be obtained 24 to 36 hours after endoscopy to rule out fistula formation. If this study is negative a repeat barium swallow should be obtained 10 to 14 days later to rule out a stricture or late-developing fistula.

Once the battery has passed through the stomach, it will usually pass without difficulty. Daily radiographs should be obtained and if the battery remains in one location longer than 36 to 48 hours or if the patient becomes symptomatic with abdominal pain or signs of perforation it should be removed via surgery.

Case reports of the use of H_2 blockers and laxatives have been reported, but neither of these treatments has proven beneficial. Emetics can lead to retrograde migration of gastric batteries into the esophagus and should be avoided.

Sharp, pointed, and elongated objects
The most common sharp and pointed objects ingested are toothpicks, nails, needles, bones, razor blades, safety pins, and dental prostheses. Often removal of these objects requires surgical intervention. In fact toothpicks and bones

are the most common foreign bodies requiring surgery.

Perforation is more likely to occur with sharp, pointed, and elongated foreign bodies than with blunter shapes. Toothpicks are prone to penetration of the gastrointestinal wall leading to complications in nearby structures, and should be removed from the esophagus or stomach even if they are not impacted. Most long foreign objects, 5 cm or longer, may pass through the esophagus or stomach but will get lodged in the retroperitoneal portion of the duodenum and result in perforation. The risk of such complications may be as high as 35% for sharp and pointed objects, thus these objects should be removed endoscopically from the stomach and proximal duodenum.

Many sharp foreign objects cannot be seen radiographically. Planning for endoscopic removal of sharp, pointed, or elongated objects should include a "dry run", i.e. simulating grasping a similar object with the equipment intended for use. Jackson's axiom "advancing points puncture, trailing do not" provides the basis on how to remove sharp or pointed foreign bodies. Thus, pointed foreign objects should be removed with the pointed end trailing to avoid perforation. If the object is lodged in the esophagus with the pointed end proximally the best technique is to grasp and carry the object into the stomach where it can be re-oriented with the pointed end trailing on extraction. Sharp and pointed objects should be removed with the use of an overtube. Often the use of endotracheal anesthesia is required to remove these objects as many of these patients are uncooperative. Some advocate treating these patients with intravenous antibiotics before endoscopic removal.

If these objects progress beyond the proximal duodenum daily radiographs should be obtained. Anecdotally some clinicians have suggested using bulking laxatives, i.e. fiber, to coat the sharp object while it passes through the small and large bowel, but currently no literature on this practice exists. None the less, if the object fails to progress for 3 consecutive days or if the patient becomes symptomatic with signs of perforation or luminal obstruction, surgical intervention should be planned.

Narcotic and cocaine packets Large quantities of narcotics and cocaine are smuggled into this country every day. A practice known as "body packing", swallowing wrapped drugs in plastic or latex condoms to avoid detection, has become popular. These packets can be seen radiographically 70% to 90% of the time. Rupture of a single packet can be fatal, thus no attempt to remove these packets endoscopically (from above or below) should be made. The use of emetics, lavage, enemas, stimulant laxatives, and cathartics should also be avoided because of the possibility of rupture. These patients should be observed as inpatients with frequent urine and serum drug screen to assess for leakage. Surgical intervention is indicated if intestinal obstruction or signs of suspected rupture occur.

Further reading

Brady PG. Esophageal foreign bodies. *Gastroenterol Clin North Am* 1991; 4: 691–701.

Faigel DO, Stotland BR, Kochman ML, *et al.* Device choice and experience level in endoscopic foreign object retrieval: an *in vivo* study. *Gastrointest Endosc* 1997; 45: 490–492.

Ginsberg, GG. Management of ingested foreign objects and food bolus impactions. *Gastrointest Endosc* 1995; 41: 33–38.

Longstreth GF, Longstreth KJ, Yao JF. Esophageal food impaction: epidemiology and therapy. A retrospective, observational study. *Gastrointest Endosc* 2001; 53: 193–198.

Mehta DI, Attia MW, Quintana EC, Cronan KM. Glucagon use for esophageal coin dislodgement in children: a prospective, double-blind, placebo-controlled trial. *Acad Emerg Med* 2001; 8: 200–203.

Vicari JJ, Johanson JF, Frakes JT. Outcomes of acute esophageal food impaction: success of the push technique. *Gastrointest Endosc* 2001; 53: 178–181.

Virgilis D, Weinberger JM, Fisher D, Goldberg S, Picard E, Kerem E. Vocal cord paralysis secondary to impacted esophageal foreign bodies in young children. *Pediatrics* 2001; 107: E101.

Webb WA. Management of foreign bodies of the upper gastrointestinal tract: update. *Gastrointest Endosc* 1995: 41; 39–51.

Chapter 13

Gastric Cancer, Lymphoma, and Carcinoids of the Stomach

David E. Loren and David C. Metz

CHAPTER OUTLINE

Gastric adenocarcinoma

Epidemiology

It is estimated that there will have been 21 600 new cases of gastric cancer in the US in 2002, and that 12 400 patients will have died of the disease. This is in the face of a progressive decline in gastric cancer in the US over recent decades. Despite the overall decline, there has been a recent increase in the incidence of cancers located in the proximal stomach and the gastroesophageal junction. Gastric cancer incidence is epidemic in some countries including Japan, Chile, and Costa Rica. Because the incidence in Japan is 100/100 000 a nationwide endoscopic screening program has been established. Interestingly, despite the high prevalence of disease, prognosis of patients with gastric cancer is better in Japan than in the US. Box 13.1 lists some of the important epidemiological features of gastric cancer in the US.

Gastric cancer is more common in African Americans and in men as compared to the remainder of the US population. Low socio-economic status may be an independent risk factor; however, this finding may be related to poor storage and preparation of food, as well

> **Box 13.1** Epidemiological features of gastric cancer in the US
>
> More common in males than in females (2:1)
> More common in African Americans than in Caucasians (1.5–2.5:1)
> Peak incidence occurs in the seventh and eighth decade

> **Box 13.2** Factors associated with the development of gastric cancer
>
> **Dietary**
> salted and pickled foods
> high nitrate content
> diets low in vitamins A and C
> diets low in fresh vegetables and fiber
>
> **Local factors**
> *Helicobacter pylori*
> intestinal metaplasia
> atrophic gastritis
> adenomatous/hyperplastic polyps
> history of distal gastrectomy
>
> **Genetic factors**
> familial adenomatous polyposis
> hereditary non-polyposis colon cancer
> hereditary diffuse gastric cancer
> Li–Fraumeni syndrome
> Peutz–Jehger syndrome
>
> **Other**
> smoking
> poor food storage and preparation
> low socioeconomic status

as an increased prevalence of *Helicobacter pylori* infection in this group. Additionally, the development of gastric cancer has been associated with the process of salting meats and fishes, and the dietary intake of nitrates, whereas diets high in vitamins A and C may be protective. Patients who have undergone distal gastrectomy, most commonly for benign ulcer disease, have an increased risk of developing cancer beginning 15 to 20 years after the surgery.

A genetic predisposition to gastric cancer has been recognized through familial clustering of gastric cancer, as well as in association with the hereditary non-polyposis colon cancer syndrome kindreds. The molecular contribution of E-cadherin mutations in diffuse hereditary gastric cancer is well described. In addition, the presence of pro-inflammatory cytokines, in particular interleukin-1, have been implicated in the development and spread of gastric cancer.

Animal models, as well as epidemiological associations, have suggested a major contribution of *H. pylori* gastritis to the development of gastric cancer. The pathophysiology by which infection may place an individual at increased risk of gastric adenocarcinoma is unclear. Because chronic atrophic gastritis and intestinal metaplasia have been shown to occur at sites of gastric carcinoma, there may be an induction of the inflammatory response by the bacterium, promoting carcinogenesis. Furthermore, other factors may play a role, including oxygen radicals, ascorbic acid, and interleukins. Nevertheless, a clear biologic progression from infection to malignancy has not been defined

and, importantly, eradication of the organism has not been convincingly shown to decrease the incidence of gastric malignancy. Box 13.2 summarizes factors associated with the development of gastric cancer.

Clinical features

The diagnosis of gastric cancer is usually suspected when clinical symptoms raise a suspicion of the disease. Because symptoms are often vague, or due to extension of the tumor, patients commonly have advanced-stage disease at the time of diagnosis. The most common symptoms are those of weight loss and abdominal pain. The weight loss is multi-factorial and may be due to an increased catabolic state coupled with decreased oral intake. Dysphagia due to tumors of the cardia or the gastroesophageal junction may further compound the problem. Early satiety in the case of diffusely invading tumor causing a linitis plastica may be evident. Nausea and vomiting as manifestations of gastric outlet or small bowel obstruction in the case of peritoneal disease, may further exacerbate nutritional depletion. In addition to pain and loss of weight, bleeding, whether overt or occult, may be the presenting manifestation in a minority of patients. The finding of a gastric ulcer in an elderly patient undergoing evaluation for anemia should raise the concern for gastric malignancy. Paraneoplastic manifestations including well-recognized dermatological changes of acanthosis nigricans and diffuse sebhorreic keratoses have been described. In addition, hematologic abnormalities, rheumatologic complications, and neurotoxicity have been reported.

Pathology

The most common histologic type of stomach cancer is adenocarcinoma, which accounts for the vast majority of tumors; less common types include lymphomas and tumors of the muscular wall layer. These are listed in Box 13.3. Classification according to the Lauren system into intestinal and diffuse types is based upon histolopathologic characteristics (Table 13.1). The intestinal type has distinct glands of

Box 13.3 Histology of stomach cancers
Adenocarcinoma
Lymphoma
Carcinoid
Leiomyosarcoma
Adenoacanthoma
Squamous cell carcinoma

malignant cells as compared to the infiltrating type, which has a poorly organized architecture, with small groups of cells or individual cells invading diffusely into the gastric wall. This latter form portends a worse prognosis as it metastasizes early in the course of disease.

Diagnosis and staging

The approach to diagnosis hinges upon identification of the gastric lesion, and obtaining an accurate tissue identification. Accordingly, many authorities recommend upper endoscopy with biopsy as the initial test of choice. Gastroscopy allows for inspection of mucosal lesions, as well as assessment of gastric distensibility and peristaltic function. In addition to evaluation of the stomach, upper endoscopy can identify esophageal or duodenal lesions that may account for symptoms in a given patient.

Table 13.1 Classification of gastric adenocarcinoma		
	Intestinal	Diffuse
Cellular histology	well differentiated columnar cells	poorly differentiated cells, may be signet ring cells
Architecture	glandular	small non-cohesive nests, solitary infiltrating cells
Luminal component	polypoid or protruding lesions	few luminal changes
Mural invasion	focal	extensive
Metastasis	late	early
Prognosis	good for early-stage disease	poor

Moreover, biopsy of suspected lesions is an important adjunct to visualization of the gastric wall and increases the sensitivity over endoscopy alone. Barium contrast radiography is complementary to endoscopy and can identify infiltrating lesions that may not be seen endoscopically. Thus, endoscopic evaluation and barium meal are useful in combination, and one should not supplant the other. Follow-up gastric evaluation for healing of gastric ulceration has been advocated to establish the diagnosis of gastric cancer. The utility of this approach has been questioned, as lesions identified in this manner are often incurable. Nevertheless, in appropriately selected patients who may be at increased risk, a follow-up examination may be warranted.

Early gastric cancer is a designation of gastric lesions that are confined to the mucosal layers irrespective of lymph-node status. The classification is more widely used in the Far East rather than in western countries, as the incidence of early gastric cancer is low in the west. Most intramucosal carcinomas are diagnosed through screening protocols in countries with a high incidence of gastric cancer. The intestinal histology is seen slightly more commonly in early gastric cancer than in the diffuse type.

Endoscopic ultrasound offers the ability to examine the wall layers of the gastric mucosa in detail. Thus, it is especially helpful in determining the extent of mucosal involvement, and can identify regional lymphadenopathy. Endoscopic ultrasound is the most accurate test for determining T stage and N stage. Moreover, endosonography may offer prognostic information and aid in defining treatment approaches in select patients. Finally, submucosal mural lesions such as leiomyomas, leiomyosarcomas, and lipomas can be well characterized by endoscopic ultrasound.

Cross-sectional imaging is used for the staging of lesions and dynamic computed tomography is the most commonly used modality. However, computed tomography may be inaccurate, particularly when assessing the depth of invasion of gastric lesions, as well as having a poor accuracy for identification of adenopathy and peritoneal metastasis. Nevertheless, computed tomography is the mainstay for identifying metastatic disease, particularly hepatic metastases.

Laparoscopy is a very sensitive technique for assessing the extent of disease. In particular, the procedure can identify malignant lymphadenopathy and peritoneal metastasis. Its use is limited by the invasiveness, potential for port-site metastasis and cost of the procedure.

Tables 13.2 and 13.3 list the TNM staging and clinical staging criteria for gastric adenocarcinoma.

Modes of spread

Gastric carcinoma may spread by local, lymphatic, or hematogenous routes. Tumors

---

Table 13.2 TNM staging for gastric adenocarcinoma

Primary tumor

TX	primary tumor cannot be assessed
T0	no evidence of primary tumor
Tis	carcinoma *in situ*
T1	invades lamina propria or submucosa
T2	invades muscularis propria
T3	invades adventitia
T4	invades adjacent structures

Regional lymph nodes

NX	regional nodes cannot be assessed
N0	no regional node involvement
N1	perigastric nodes within 3 cm of tumor margin
N2	perigastric nodes more than 3 cm from tumor margin, nodes along left gastric, common hepatic, splenic, or celiac arteries

Distant metastasis

MX	distant metastasis cannot be assessed
M0	no distant metastasis
M1	distant metastasis

Table 13.3 Clinical staging for gastric adenocarcinoma

Stage 0	Tis, N0, M0
Stage IA	T1, N0, M0
Stage IB	T1, N1, M0
	T2, N0, M0
Stage II	T1, N2, M0
	T2, N1, M0
	T3, N0, M0
Stage IIIA	T2, N2, M0
	T3, N1, M0
	T4, N0, M0
Stage IIIB	T3, N2, M0
	T4, N1, M0
Stage IV	T4, N2, M0
	Any T, any N, M1

extend from their site of origin into the gastric wall and expand, thus involving greater portions of the stomach. This type of spread may be superficial only, or it may involve deeper wall layers extending to the esophagus or duodenum. Local tumor growth may progress further into adjacent organs or the peritoneum, which results in peritoneal carcinomatosis. Lymph–node metastasis occurs locoregionally in relation to the anatomic site of the tumor, and may then extend along the perigastric, splenic, hepatoduodenal, or celiac nodal chains. Classic findings for intraabdominal carcinomatosis include Virchow's node (left supraclavicular adenopathy), Sister Mary Joseph's node (periumbilical palpable node), Krukenberg's tumor (ovarian metastasis) and Blummer's shelf (palpable metastasis in the peritoneal cul-de-sac). Distant spread occurs to the liver most commonly, followed by peritoneal and mesenteric metastasis. Osseous, pulmonary, pancreatic, and adrenal metastasis are other locations of distant spread. Accordingly, staging of patients should include not only local evaluation, but also computed tomography of the chest, abdomen, and pelvis to identify metastatic sites.

Management

Curative surgery

Complete resection of the tumor is the mainstay of treatment when the goal is to achieve cure of the disease. Unfortunately, two thirds of patients in the US are diagnosed with incurable disease (stages II or III). The extent of tumor and local lymphadenopathy are the primary determinants of choice of resection. For intramucosal carcinoma, endoscopic mucosal resection has become an increasingly performed procedure in select patients. Careful staging by endoscopy and endoscopic ultrasound are mandatory prior to performing this limited excision. Total versus subtotal gastrectomy are the transabdominal procedures performed with curative intent. Distal cancers may be more amenable to a subtotal approach compared to proximal lesions. A proximal subtotal gastrectomy can be performed for cases of proximal lesions that do not involve the gastroesophageal junction. Even in the absence of demonstrable unresectability, the finding of linitis plastica is considered to be a contraindication to surgery as prognosis is very poor and the benefit of surgery in this setting has not been demonstrated. A debated issue is the benefit of performing an extensive lymphadenectomy that may include splenectomy. In Japan, where an extended lymphadenectomy is commonly performed, the procedure offers more precise staging, and improved stage-specific management. However, the added morbidity of this procedure limits its application and the benefits of the procedure in management have not been conclusively determined. Table 13.4 lists the surgical procedures of choice appropriate to the anatomic site of the primary tumor.

Palliative interventions

Patients with unresectable carcinoma may require surgery for palliation of local

Table 13.4 Surgical procedures of choice for resection of gastric adenocarcinoma

Site of tumor	Choice of procedure
Intramucosal carcinoma	endoscopic mucosal resection versus subtotal gastrectomy
Gastroesophageal junction	distal esophagectomy, subtotal proximal gastrectomy with gastric pull through
Proximal Stomach	subtotal proximal gastrectomy versus total gastrectomy
Distal stomach	subtotal gastrectomy

complications or for management of metastatic disease. Complications that may be best treated surgically include intractable nausea, intestinal obstruction, recurrent bleeding, and aspiration. Palliative gastrectomy may be performed to control bleeding, pain, and nausea, or to relieve obstruction, and consists of a total gastrectomy with esophagojejunostomy. In cases where the stomach cannot be adequately removed a bypass procedure may be performed. While palliative surgeries can generally control the immediate complications of gastric cancer, it is debated whether there is an improvement in survival or quality of life. Accordingly, the decision to perform a palliative procedure is an individualized process taking into account the surgical feasibility, potential benefits of the procedure, surgical risks, and patient preferences.

Increasingly, endoscopic management of tumor complications is used to avoid major surgery in patients who have incurable disease. This approach is offered frequently as many patients are often not suitable for operations either because of malnutrition, concurrent medical problems, or advancing age. Enteral stenting is the placement of expandable prostheses into the lumen of the gastrointestinal tract to relieve obstruction. Additionally, endoscopic techniques may be employed to manage bleeding complications or to perform a gastrostomy to allow for gastric venting in the obstructed patient. Endoscopic or surgical jejunostomy can allow for enteral feeding when gastric obstruction precludes oral or gastrostomy tube feeding.

Radiotherapy

Gastric adenocarcinoma is generally resistant to external beam radiation. Numerous trials have investigated the use of neoadjuvant, intraoperative, and postoperative use of radiotherapy. The majority of the studies are confounded by a lack of control groups, disparity in outcome measures, variability in the surgeries performed, and differences in the diagnostic and management patterns of areas with high prevalence versus low prevalence of disease. Accordingly, there is no generally accepted standard for the administration of radiotherapy for gastric cancer, although there are scant data on radiation alone for palliation to manage complications of obstruction, bleeding or pain.

Chemotherapy

Systemic chemotherapy has been associated with, at best, a moderate improvement in survival for patients with gastric cancer undergoing surgery. The benefit may be greater for those with disease metastatic to the lymph nodes compared to individuals with disease confined to the stomach. In a large proportion of cases, adverse effects from the therapy limit the ability of patients to receive a full course of medication. The most common use of chemotherapy for patients with potentially resectable disease is in combination with radiation as it serves as a radiosensitizer to enhance the effects or radiotherapy.

For those with advanced cancer, for whom curative surgery is not an option but who have a good performance status, the standard therapy is epirubicin, cisplatin, and 5-fluorouracil in combination. This regimen offers a response rate of 45% and a median survival of nine months.

Combination chemoradiation

The use of combination chemoradiation in the postoperative setting has yielded mixed results and thus postoperative therapy should be considered in the context of clinical trials whenever possible. A recent study of more than 500 patients with adenocarcinoma of the gastroesophageal junction and gastric cardia supported a benefit to multimodal therapy using fluorouracil and leucovorin in combination with radiotherapy. The results of this study may significantly impact the management of patients with gastroesophageal junction tumors.

Clinical course and prognosis

The pathologic staging of gastric cancer is the most important determinant of survival. For those with stage 0 disease (carcinoma in situ) 5-year survival exceeds 90%, and stage I patients have a 60% to 80% survival at 5 years. Unfortunately, most patients in the US are diagnosed with stage III or IV disease that carries a 5-year survival of less than 20% and 10% respectively. Other poor prognostic features include the diffuse type of cancer (as compared to intestinal), poorly differentiated tumors, and more proximal lesions. Molecular markers offer prognostic significance as those with aneuploid tumors, and tumors with aberrations in oncogenes or tumor suppressor genes tend to have a worse prognosis. These findings are more common in North American patients with gastric cancer who tend to fare worse than those in countries with a higher incidence of gastric cancer.

Figure 13.1 is an algorithm for the diagnosis and management of patients with suspected gastric adenocarcinoma.

Gastric lymphoma

Primary lymphomatous involvement of the gastrointestinal tract is an uncommon event; however, the stomach is the most common location for primary lesions. In contrast, the gastrointestinal tract is the extranodal location most often affected by spread of nodal-based disease, occurring in up to 60% of patients. Both Hodgkin's and Non-Hodgkin's lymphoma may present with primary gastric lesions, the latter accounting for the vast majority of cases. The most common subtypes of gastric non-Hodgkin's lymphoma are those arising in the setting of mucosal-associated lymphoid tissue (see Classification on p. 191). Other non-Hodgkin's lymphoma subtypes include Mantle cell lymphoma, Burkitt's lymphoma, and follicular lymphoma. Hodgkin's disease of the gastrointestinal tract is exceedingly rare whether as a primary lesion or present along with other sites of disease.

Epidemiology

Gastric lymphoma generally develops in the fifth decade of life and occurs more commonly in men than women. The most frequent presenting symptom is abdominal pain, although fevers and weight loss, night sweats, anorexia, early satiety, nausea, or bleeding may be present. Anemia may transpire due to poor nutritional status, malabsorption of macronutrients, or blood loss.

There are data to suggest an increase in the incidence of gastrointestinal non-Hodgkin's lymphoma over recent decades; the cause of this increase is unclear. In part this may be

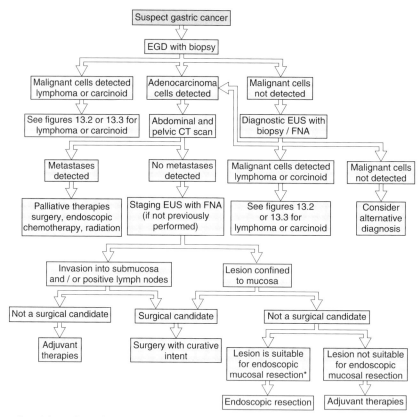

Figure 13.1 Algorithm for the evaluation and treatment of suspected gastric cancer. EGD esophagogastricduodenoscopy; CT computed tomography; FNA fine-needle aspiration; EUS endoscopic ultrasound; * less than 2 cm, no ulceration of lesion.

due to increased detection because of increased screening in the *Helicobacter pylori* era. Risk factors for the development of gastric lymphoma are infection with *H. pylori*, autoimmune disorders such as Hashimoto's thyroiditis or Sjogren's disease, and the presence of immunosuppression, either congenital or acquired due to HIV or medications. There is a clear association between *H. pylori* infection and the mucosal-associated lymphoid tissue (MALT) type of gastric lymphoma. In this setting, the eradication of *H. pylori* alone may be the only treatment recommended for those with early stage disease. The presence of inflammatory bowel disease has been thought to place an individual at increased risk, but this may be more a result of the immunosuppressive therapies used for

these patients, than the underlying bowel process.

Diagnosis

The diagnostic procedure of choice for a patient in whom a gastric lymphoma is suspected is upper endoscopy with biopsy, which can make the histologic diagnosis in greater than 90% of cases. Direct visualization and sampling of a lesion allows for an assessment not only of the extent of disease, but also for the histologic characterization necessary for accurate classification. Gastric findings of a multinodular appearance, thickened gastric folds, or a frank mass raise concerns of a gastric lymphoma. Barium radiography is less sensitive in detecting abnormalities, but may identify mucosal abnormalities approximately 70% of the time.

Classification

Advances in our understanding of the clinical behavior and molecular features of non–Hodgkin's lymphoma have resulted in an evo-

lution in the classification systems. The World Health Organization has advocated the use of the Revised European American Lymphoma (REAL) system (Table 13.5). The basis for this categorization is the aggressiveness of the clinical behavior of the lymphoma as determined by survival data, coupled with histopathologic and molecular features. This classification scheme provides for inclusion of lymphoma subtypes not accounted for in other classification systems. In this format the MALT lymphoma is designated as either the indolent 'extranodal marginal zone B-cell lymphoma' or the more aggressive diffuse large B-cell lymphoma.

Upon obtaining tissue, lesions are evaluated for histologic diagnosis and immunophenotyping is performed. Extranodal marginal B-cell lymphoma appears as a collection of small lymphocytes, marginal zone B cells which infiltrate the epithelium, monocytoid B cells, plasma cells, and large basophilic immunoblast-like cells. The lesion generally arises within an area of reactive lymphoid follicles. Diffuse large B-cell lymphoma can have a varied histologic appearance, but most commonly is a mixture of immunoblast- and centroblast-like cells. Follicular lymphomas are comprised of mainly follicle cells, whereas the malignant cell in Mantle cell lymphoma is located around germinal centers, and occurs either as an aggressive form similar to Burkitt's lymphoma or a more benign phenotype. Burkitt's lymphoma is an extremely aggressive lymphoma, which is histologically composed of medium-sized cells, often multinucleated, with a high mitotic index. Importantly, for accurate characterization of the lymphoma subtype, molecular marker profiles based on flow cytometry are complementary to the histologic appearance.

Table 13.5 Revised European American lymphoma (REAL) classification system for non-Hodgkin's lymphoma

Indolent lymphomas
B-cell
   small lymphocytic lymphoma/B-cell chronic
     lymphocytic leukemia
   lymphoplasmacytoid lymphoma
   plasma cell myeloma/plasmacytoma
   hairy cell leukemia
   follicular lymphoma (grade I & II)[*]
   marginal zone lymphoma[*]
   Mantle cell lymphoma[*]
T-cell
   T-cell large granular lymphocyte leukemia
     mycosis fungoides
   T-cell promyelocytic leukemia natural
     killer-cell
   natural killer-cell large granular
     lymphocytic leukemia

Aggressive lymphomas
follicular lymphoma (grade III)[*]
diffuse large B-cell lymphoma[*]
peripheral T-cell lymphoma
anaplastic large cell lymphoma

Highly aggressive lymphomas
Burkitt's lymphoma[*]
precursor B lymphoblastic leukemia/
  lymphoma
adult T-cell lymphoma/leukemia
precursor T-cell
  lymphoblasticlymphoma/leukemia

[*]lymphomas occurring as primary gastric lesions.

Staging

Staging evaluation for individuals diagnosed with gastric lymphoma should include a

Table 13.6 Staging of gastric non-Hodgkin's lymphoma		
Stage I	tumor confined to the stomach	I_1 Infiltration of the mucosa and/or submucosa. I_2 Infiltration into muscularis and/or subserosa and/or serosa, does not extend to adjacent tissues.
Stage II	tumor extends into abdomen from primary gastric site	II_1 Local extension to perigastric nodes. II_2 Distant nodal involvement of mesenteric, para-aortic, paracaval, pelvic, or inguinal nodes.
Stage III	tumor penetrates serosa into adjacent tissues and organs	$III_{[pancreas]}$, $III_{[colon]}$, $III_{[postabdominal wall]}$.
Stage IV	disseminated extranodal involvement	Involvement of bone marrow or liver. Also includes supra-diaphramatic nodal disease.

cross-sectional evaluation of the chest, abdomen, and pelvis. This is most often performed with computed tomography. In addition, gastric endoscopic ultrasound should be performed for determining the depth of penetration of the lesion, as well as for assessment of regional lymphadenopathy. Fine-needle aspiration of perigastric lymph nodes may be performed to enhance the specificity of the endosonographic examination. In select cases, a diagnostic laparoscopy or laparotomy may be performed to complete the staging. Local staging involves assessment of depth of tumor invasion, nodal assessment involvement of adjacent organs, and disseminated disease (Table 13.6).

Management

Indolent lymphomas

Extranodal marginal zone B-cell lymphoma, also known as gastric MALT lymphoma, presents most often as an isolated gastric lesion, although multiple sites of disease can be found in up to 20% of cases. This lesion is strongly associated with the presence of *Helicobacter pylori* infection, and eradication of the organism may be sufficient therapy in selected patients. Patients who may benefit from this approach are those with low-grade histology, and disease confined to the mucosa as determined by endoscopic ultrasound. More aggressive therapies, including surgery and adjuvant chemotherapy, are required for those who do not respond to *H. pylori* eradication. Additionally, more extensive tumors that invade the gastric wall or involve perigastric lymph nodes, as well as those with high-grade histologic findings, should undergo *H. pylori* eradication along with more aggressive therapies. Regarding other low-grade gastric B cell lymphomas, approaches may include chemotherapy, radiation, and surgical modalities depending upon the tumor subtype and stage at the time of diagnosis. In these cases, management decisions are made on an individualized basis.

Aggressive lymphomas

The high-grade histology associated with MALT is diffuse large B-cell lymphoma. This lesion may be found on gastric biopsy or in those who initially carry a diagnosis of low-grade disease but do not respond to *Helicobacter pylori* eradication, and undergo subsequent gastrectomy, at which time diffuse large B-cell lymphoma may be found. Surgery is offered for diffuse large B-cell lymphoma when confined to the stomach or when adjacent lymph nodes are involved. For more extensive disease there is little role for resection. Burkitt's lymphoma usually presents with late-stage disease because of its aggressive nature, and systemic therapy is invariably necessary. In a minority of cases, cure may be achieved with aggressive chemotherapy.

Figure 13.2 shows an algorithm for the diagnosis and management of suspected gastric lymphoma.

Gastric carcinoid tumors

Carcinoid tumors are the most common neuroendocrine tumor affecting the alimentary tract, with the stomach being an uncommon site, accounting for only 2% to 3% of all carcinoid tumors. Carcinoid tumors received their name because of their slow-growing nature, thus being similar to a carcinoma, but behaving in a more indolent fashion.

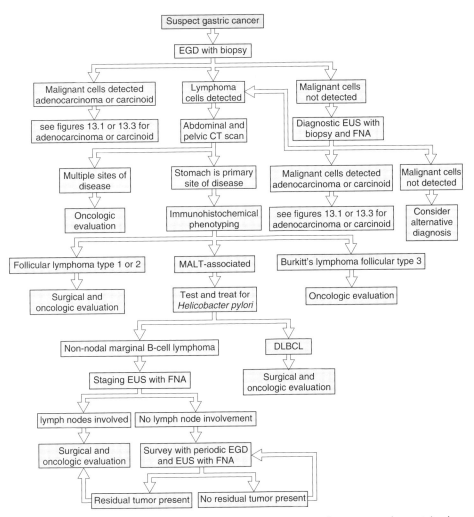

Figure 13.2 Evaluation for the evaluation and treatment of suspected gastric lymphoma. EGD esophagogastricduodenoscopy; CT computed tomography; FNA fine-needle aspiration; EUS endoscopic ultrasound; MALT mucosal-associated lymphoid tissue; DLBCL diffuse large-cell B-cell lymphoma.

Classification

Carcinoid tumors can generally be classified according to their site of embryonal origin into foregut, midgut, and hindgut, with gastric tumors being foregut lesions. When considering gastric carcinoids, they are further classified according to the presence or absence of hypergastrinemia. Those with elevated gastrin levels are further classified according to the etiology of the gastrin hypersecretion.

Type 1 carcinoid tumors arise from ECL cells and are thus generally found in the fundus and body of the stomach. Clinically they are associated with achlorhydria due to chronic atrophic gastritis and pernicious anemia. This results in a hypergastrinemic state due to the absence of acid production and subsequent loss of feedback inhibition of gastrin production. While the pathophysiology is thought to be due to stimulation of gastrin on the ECL cells, local and systemic mediators may play a role, particularly inflammatory cytokines. Patients are usually found to have multiple lesions at the time of diagnosis; however, their clinical course is less aggressive than other gastric carcinoids. Nevertheless, metastasis and its attendant morbidity and mortality may transpire. Type 1 lesions are the most common type of gastric carcinoid tumor.

Type 2 carcinoids arise in the setting of hypergastrinemia due to Zollinger–Ellison syndrome. These account for approximately 5% of gastric carcinoids. Similarities to type 1 carcinoids include the presence of hypergastrinemia, the ECL cell as the cell of origin, the presence of multiple lesions at the time of diagnosis, and a generally indolent course. Inactivation at the MEN-1 gene locus is found in the majority of type 2 tumors.

Type 3 tumors, also known as sporadic carcinoids, do not occur in a hypergastrinemic state. They are usually single, large lesions with an aggressive course with metastases present at the time of diagnosis. Type 3 lesions may present with the carcinoid syndrome, unlike type 1 or 2 where the clinical carcinoid syndrome does not generally occur.

Table 13.7 illustrates the features of the various types of carcinoid tumors.

Clinical features

Carcinoid tumors are most often found incidentally during evaluation for unrelated problems. When symptoms do occur, they may be related to the tumor itself, the presence of the carcinoid syndrome, or the underlying hypergastrinemic state. Abdominal pain, upper gastrointestinal bleeding, diarrhea, nausea, and vomiting are common symptoms, whereas flushing, bronchospasm and diarrhea occur less often. The carcinoid syndrome may occur in 5% of patients with gastric carcinoids; however, because the hormonal product of

Table 13.7 Classification of gastric carcinoid tumors

Classification	Presence of hypergastrinemia	Underlying disease associations	Number of lesions
Type 1	yes	chronic atrophic gastritis pernicious anemia	multiple
Type 2	yes	Zollinger–Ellison syndrome multiple endocrine neoplasia type 1	multiple
Type 3	no	carcinoid syndrome	single

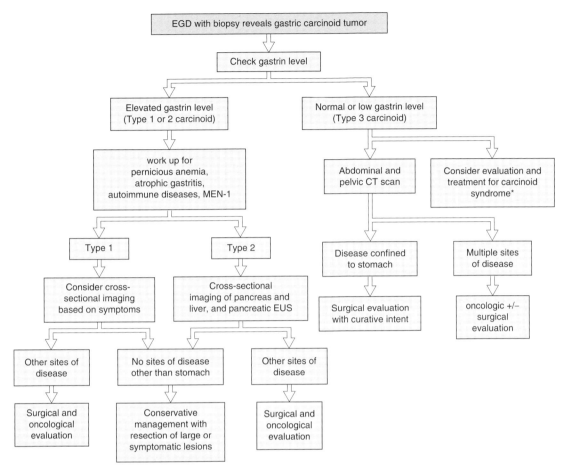

Figure 13.3 Algorithm for the evaluation and treatment of gastric carcinoid tumors. EGD esophagogastricduodenoscopy; MEN-1 multiple endocrine neoplasia type 1; EUS endoscopic ultrasound;
* evaluation may include urine 5-HIAA and 5-HTP, serum histamine and serotonin, somatostatin receptor scintigraphy.

gastric tumors is more often histamine rather than serotonin, the features of the syndrome are considered to be atypical. The atypical syndrome consists of violaceous flushing and bronchospasm without diarrhea, occurring in a sustained fashion. This is in contrast to the classic intermittent symptoms of hypotension, flushing, and diarrhea seen in midgut tumors when lesions have metastasized to the liver. Cardiac valvular disease is uncommon in patients with tumors isolated to the stomach, but when it does occur it tends to involve the left side of the heart.

Diagnosis

The diagnosis of gastric carcinoid may be made during evaluation for symptoms localized to the abdomen, concerns of a hormonally functional syndrome, or as an incidental finding. Upper endoscopy may identify visible lesions of single or multiple masses, ulcers, and thickened folds related to the Zollinger–Ellison syndrome, or the flattened mucosa of atrophic gastritis. Gastric acidity can be determined at the time of endoscopy to assist in evaluation of a hypergastrinemic state. Hormonal evaluation can be performed with analysis of urine for 5-hydroxyindoleacetic acid, the breakdown product of serotonin, or the serotonin precursor 5-hydroxytryptophan. Serum levels of serotonin, 5-hydroxytryptophan, chromogranin, and histamine can be measured. Somatostatin-receptor scintigraphy has a sensitivity of 75% in patients with Zollinger–Ellison syndrome although for initial diagnostic purposes, its utility is questionable.

Upon diagnosis of a carcinoid tumor, staging should be performed with endoscopic ultrasound for local tumor and lymph-node staging, as well as cross-sectional imaging to identify metastases.

Management

The symptoms of patients suffering from carcinoid syndrome may respond to treatment with somatostatin analogues. However, while medical management may control symptoms, it is not effective therapy for tumor control.

Tumor excision is the treatment modality of choice for gastric carcinoid tumors, and the method of excision varies according to type of gastric carcinoid and size of the tumor. Endoscopic removal may be considered in selected patient whose carcinoids are related to a hypergastrinemic state (types 1 and 2). For these patients, carcinoids that are less than 2 cm in size and confined to the mucosa and submucosa, as determined endosonographically, may undergo endoscopic excision. If lesions are invasive or larger than 2 cm in size, surgical resection is advised. For superficial lesions 1 to 2 cm in size, optimal management strategies are controversial. Type 3 gastric carcinoids should be removed surgically along with lymph-node resection, as these tumors are more aggressive and are often invasive at the time of diagnosis.

In the case of metastatic disease, therapies are limited. Chemotherapy as single agent or in combination does not offer a significant benefit. Tumor-directed therapies such as hepatic

resection, arterial chemoembolization, and radiation-emitting somatostatin receptor analogues may offer a temporizing response and are under investigation.

Figure 13.3 illustrates an algorithm for the diagnosis and management of gastric carcinoid tumors.

Further reading

Bonenkamp JJ, Hermans J, Sasako M, van de Velde CJ. Extended lymph-node dissection for gastric cancer. Dutch Gastric Cancer Group. *N Engl J Med* 1999; 340(12): 908–914.

Crump M, Gospodarowicz M, Shepherd FA. Lymphoma of the gastrointestinal tract. *Semin Oncol* 1999; 26(3): 324–337.

Cuschieri A, Weeden S, Fielding J, *et al.* Patient survival after D1 and D2 resections for gastric cancer: long-term results of the MRC randomized surgical trial. Surgical Co-operative Group. *Br J Cancer* 1999; 79(9–10): 1522–1530.

El-Omar EM, Carrington M, Chow WH, *et al.* Interleukin-1 polymorphisms associated with increased risk of gastric cancer. *Nature* 2000; 404(6776): 398–402.

Feldman RA. Review article: would eradication of *Helicobacter pylori* infection reduce the risk of gastric cancer? *Aliment Pharmacol Ther* 2001; 15 (suppl. 1): 2–5.

Fuchs CS, Mayer RJ. Gastric carcinoma. *N Engl J Med* 1995; 333(1): 32–41.

Granberg D, Wilander E, Stridsberg M, Granerus G, Skogseid B, Oberg K. Clinical symptoms, hormone profiles, treatment, and prognosis in patients with gastric carcinoids. *Gut* 1998; 43(2): 223–228.

Grimm H, Binmoeller KF, Hamper K, Koch J, Henne-Bruns D, Soehendra N. Endosonography for preoperative locoregional staging of esophageal and gastric cancer. *Endoscopy* 1993; 25(3): 224–230.

Guilford PJ, Hopkins JB, Grady WM, *et al.* E-cadherin germline mutations define an inherited cancer syndrome dominated by diffuse gastric cancer. *Hum Mutat* 1999; 14(3): 249–255.

Hanazaki K, Sodeyama H, Mochizuki Y, *et al.* Palliative gastrectomy for advanced gastric cancer. *Hepatogastroenterology* 2001; 48(37): 285–289.

Jemal A, Thomas A, Murray T, Thun M. Cancer statistics, 2002. *CA Cancer J Clin* 2002; 52(1): 23–47.

Levy M, Copie-Bergman C, Traulle C, *et al.* Conservative treatment of primary gastric low-grade B-cell lymphoma of mucosa-associated lymphoid tissue: predictive factors of response and outcome. *Am J Gastroenterol* 2002; 97(2): 292–297.

Macdonald JS, Smalley SR, Benedetti J, *et al.* Chemoradiotherapy after surgery compared with surgery alone for adenocarcinoma of the stomach or gastroesophageal junction. *N Engl J Med* 2001; 345(10): 725–730.

Pruitt RE, Truss CD. Endoscopy, gastric ulcer, and gastric cancer. Follow-up endoscopy for all gastric ulcers? *Dig Dis Sci* 1993; 38(2): 284–288.

Uemura N, Okamoto S, Yamamoto S, *et al. Helicobacter pylori* infection and the development of gastric cancer. *N Engl J Med* 2001; 345(11): 784–789.

Index